Burning Calories
Made Simple

A Practical Guide to Effective Weight Loss and Transformation of Your Body

Table of Contents

Introduction:

The Sane Solution to Weight Loss and Transformation

Let's be honest: weight loss is often made to seem way more complicated than it needs to be. Every day, we're bombarded with quick fixes, magic pills, or extreme diets that promise transformation but rarely deliver long-term results. No wonder so many people feel frustrated, stuck, and ready to throw in the towel.

But here's the truth: weight loss doesn't have to be an endless cycle of misery, restriction, and confusion. It can be simple, sustainable, and—believe it or not—enjoyable. That's what this book is about. This is the sane solution to weight loss.

The Power of Understanding Calories

At the heart of this approach is something so basic that it's often overlooked: calories. But knowing your calories is more than just reading numbers on a label. When you understand how they work, you gain control over your health, your energy, and your weight.

Think of calories as the currency of energy. You spend them when you move, you consume them when you eat, and your body stores or burns them based on how much you have in the bank. Understanding this simple concept can unlock the door to achieving your goals without feeling like you're punishing yourself every day.

Knowing your calories allows you to make informed choices rather than guessing. Instead of feeling powerless, you'll discover that you can tweak small things in your daily routine and see big results. Whether you're just starting out or you've tried every diet in the book, understanding calories can change everything.

Transform Your Body, Elevate Your Life

Weight loss and body transformation aren't just about looking different—they're about living differently. By focusing on burning calories in a way that works for your life, you can shed the frustration that comes with yo-yo diets and quick-fix solutions. You can start to enjoy the process of becoming the best version of yourself, both inside and out.

This journey isn't about perfection. It's about progress. Imagine what life would feel like with more energy, greater confidence, and the ability to fully enjoy the things that matter most. That's the real benefit of taking control of your health. It's not just about the number on the scale; it's about improving the quality of your life in every way.

As you go through the chapters in this book, you'll discover practical ways to burn calories that fit into your life—whether it's through mindful eating, simple exercises, or everyday activities. You'll learn how to set yourself up for success with strategies that make sense and habits that stick. And best of all, you'll realize that you can do this.

This is about embracing a lifestyle that transforms your body and mind. It's about showing yourself that the sane solution is the one that works—and keeps working.

Welcome to your transformation.

Chapter 1: Understanding Calories and How They Affect Weight

WHAT ARE CALORIES?

Calories might seem like a mystery, but they're actually quite simple when you break it down. At their core, calories are a measure of energy—just like how miles measure distance or liters measure volume. They represent the energy your body gets from food and drinks and the energy it uses for everything you do, from breathing and thinking to running and lifting weights.

Calories: The Energy Unit of the Body

Think of a calorie as a unit of fuel. Your body is like an engine, constantly running and requiring energy to function. Whether you're sitting at your desk, going for a jog, or even sleeping, your body is always burning calories to keep your systems running smoothly. Every movement you make and every thought you have requires energy. That's what calories are for—they're the fuel that keeps you going.

But it's not just about movement. Your body uses calories for all sorts of processes: digesting food, repairing cells, circulating blood, and even regulating your body temperature. You even burn calories while you sleep. This energy is essential for everything you do, no matter how small or large the activity.

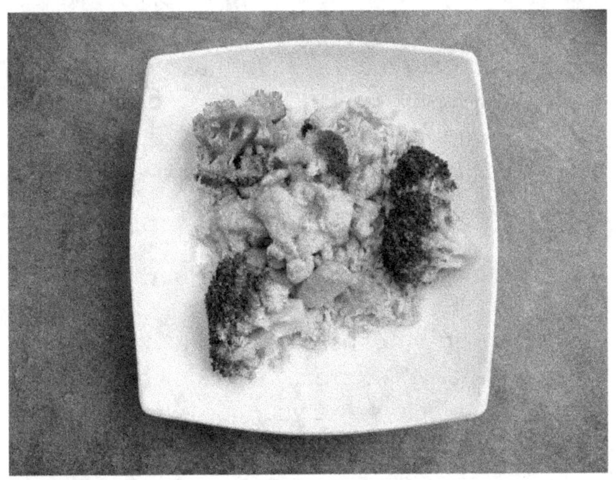

Calories in Food: How they are Measured

Now, when it comes to the food you eat, every item contains a specific number of calories. These are listed on food labels, and they represent how much energy your body can extract from that food. Foods get their calories from three main sources: carbohydrates, proteins, and fats. Each of these nutrients provides a different amount of energy:

- Carbohydrates: 4 calories per gram
- Protein: 4 calories per gram

- Fat: 9 calories per gram

This is why high-fat foods tend to be more calorie-dense, while foods rich in fiber or water, like fruits and vegetables, are lower in calories. By understanding how calories are measured in food, you gain the power to make choices that align with your goals. You can adjust portion sizes, swap ingredients, and know exactly what you're fueling your body with—no more guessing.

Estimating your Daily Energy Needs

So, how do you know how many calories you need in a day? Your daily caloric needs depend on several factors, like your age, weight, activity level, and even your metabolism. The total number of calories your body uses in a day is often referred to as your *Total Daily Energy Expenditure* (TDEE). This includes:

1. Basal Metabolic Rate (BMR): The calories you burn at rest, just keeping your body alive.
2. Physical Activity: The energy used for all movement, from walking to working out.
3. Thermic Effect of Food (TEF): The energy used to digest and process what you eat.

To get a rough estimate of how many calories you need each day, you can use simple online calculators or formulas that take into account your age, gender, weight, height, and activity level. But remember, these numbers are just estimates. Your true caloric needs may vary slightly based on factors like muscle mass and overall health.

Understanding calories isn't about restricting yourself—it's about knowing how much energy your body needs to thrive. Once you know your daily needs, you can make adjustments to either lose, maintain, or gain weight, depending on your goals.

This knowledge gives you control and confidence, empowering you to fuel your body with what it needs for optimal health and energy.

The Role of Calories in Weight Management

When it comes to weight management, calories play a central role. At the most basic level, it all comes down to the balance between the calories you consume and the calories you burn. This is often referred to as *calories in versus calories out*, and understanding this equation is the foundation for effective weight management.

The concept is straightforward: if you take in more calories than your body uses (calories in), the excess gets stored as fat, leading to weight gain. On the flip side, if you consume fewer calories than your body burns (calories out), your body taps into its energy reserves—usually stored fat—and you lose weight.

It might sound overly simplistic, but this energy balance is the key to understanding weight management. If you consistently eat more than your body needs, the extra energy has to go somewhere, and that somewhere is typically your fat stores. If you eat less than you burn, your body has no choice but to use the energy it's stored, leading to weight loss.

Energy Balance: What Happens When You Eat More or Fewer Calories

Your body is constantly seeking a state of balance, also known as *homeostasis*. When you eat the exact amount of calories your body needs, you maintain your current weight—this is called *energy balance*.

But when you eat more or fewer calories than your body requires, the balance shifts:

- **Caloric surplus** (eating more than you burn): Your body stores the extra energy as fat, leading to weight gain.
- **Caloric deficit** (eating fewer than you burn): Your body turns to stored fat for energy, resulting in weight loss.

This doesn't mean you need to aim for perfection every single day. Weight gain or loss happens gradually, over time, depending on whether you're in a surplus or deficit. If you overeat occasionally, it won't instantly cause significant weight gain, just as one day of eating less won't instantly make you lose weight. It's the long-term patterns that matter most.

Misconceptions about Calorie Counting

While calorie counting can be a helpful tool for managing your weight, it's often misunderstood. One common misconception is that all calories are created equal. Technically, a calorie is a calorie, whether it comes from broccoli or a cookie. But the way your body processes different types of food varies. Whole foods like fruits, vegetables, lean proteins, and whole grains provide more than just calories—they offer vital nutrients that help your body function at its best.

On the other hand, highly processed foods might have the same number of calories, but they don't offer the same nutritional value. They're often low in fiber and nutrients, which can leave you feeling hungry or unsatisfied, making it harder to stick to your goals. So, while the number of calories is important, the *quality* of those calories matters, too.

Another misconception is that calorie counting is too restrictive or tedious. In reality, it doesn't have to be about obsessing over every bite. It's about awareness—knowing roughly how much you're consuming and how it aligns with your goals. With practice, this can become second nature, and many people find that they don't need to count every calorie to maintain their progress. Instead, they develop a better understanding of portion sizes and food choices.

In the end, calories are a tool, not the enemy. Understanding how they work and how to balance them with your daily energy needs can empower you to manage your weight in a way that feels sustainable and manageable for the long term. It's not about restriction—it's about finding a balance that works for you.

How to Calculate your Calorie Needs

Knowing how many calories your body needs each day is the first step toward effectively managing your weight. It's not a one-size-fits-all number; instead, your calorie needs are influenced by factors like your age, weight, activity level, and even how your body functions at rest. To get an accurate idea of your daily calorie requirements, let's break it down into two key components: *Basal Metabolic Rate (BMR)* and *Total Daily Energy Expenditure (TDEE).*

Basal Metabolic Rate (BMR): What It Is And How To Calculate It

Your Basal Metabolic Rate (BMR) is the number of calories your body needs to perform basic functions like breathing, circulating blood, and regulating body temperature while at complete rest. Even if you were to lie in bed all day, your body would still need a certain amount of energy just to keep you alive. This is your BMR.

Several factors influence your BMR, including your age, gender, weight, height, and muscle mass. People with more muscle generally have higher BMRs because muscle tissue burns more calories than fat, even at rest.

To calculate your BMR, you can use the **Mifflin-St Jeor Equation**, one of the most widely used formulas:

For men:-

$$BMR = 10 \times \text{weight in kg} + 6.25 \times \text{height in cm} - 5 \times \text{age in years} + 5$$

For women:-

BMR=10×weight in kg+6.25×height in cm−5×age in years−161BMR = 10 \times \text{weight in kg} + 6.25 \times \text{height in cm} - 5 \times \text{age in years} - 161BMR=10×weight in kg+6.25×height in cm−5×age in years−161

Once you know your BMR, you have a starting point. But remember, your body doesn't just burn calories at rest—there's more to the picture.

Total Daily Energy Expenditure (TDEE): The Factors that Influence It

Your *Total Daily Energy Expenditure (TDEE)* is a more complete picture of your daily calorie needs because it accounts for all the activities you do throughout the day, from walking and exercising to eating and digesting food. TDEE includes your BMR plus the energy you burn through:

1. **Physical Activity:** This ranges from light movement, like walking or doing household chores, to more intense workouts or sports.
2. **Thermic Effect of Food (TEF):** The energy your body uses to digest, absorb, and process the food you eat.

This accounts for about 10% of your total calorie burn.

3. **Non-Exercise Activity Thermogenesis (NEAT):** The calories burned through everyday activities like fidgeting, standing, or taking the stairs.

To estimate your TDEE, you multiply your BMR by an activity factor that corresponds to your lifestyle. Here's a rough guide:

- **Sedentary (little to no exercise):** BMR × 1.2
- **Lightly active (light exercise or sports 1-3 days a week):** BMR × 1.375
- **Moderately active (moderate exercise or sports 3-5 days a week):** BMR × 1.55
- **Very active (hard exercise 6-7 days a week):** BMR × 1.725
- **Super active (very hard exercise and a physically demanding job):** BMR × 1.9

This gives you an estimate of how many calories you burn in a typical day. From there, you can adjust your intake based on whether you want to lose, maintain, or gain weight.

Online Tools and Apps for Calorie Tracking

Thankfully, you don't need to manually calculate your BMR and TDEE every day—there are plenty of online tools and apps that can do the math for you and help you stay on track. Popular apps like **MyFitnessPal**, **Lose It!**, and **Cronometer** make it easy to input your personal details, calculate your calorie needs, and track your daily intake and exercise.

These tools can also help you track macronutrients (carbs, proteins, and fats), ensuring that you're not just hitting your calorie goals but also getting a well-balanced diet. Many apps also allow you to scan barcodes, search food databases, and track your progress over time, making the process of staying aware of your calorie intake more convenient and less overwhelming.

Whether you prefer to track your calories meticulously or just use the estimates to guide your food choices, these tools provide a simple, effective way to stay in tune with your body's energy needs.

By understanding and calculating your BMR and TDEE, you gain valuable insight into how your body works and how to fuel it properly. This knowledge puts you in control of your health and weight management journey, allowing you to make informed decisions that lead to lasting results.

The Science of Fat Storage and Usage

Understanding calories is crucial to effective weight loss because they determine how your body stores and uses energy. When you consume more calories than your body needs, it stores the excess as fat. On the other hand, when you take in fewer calories than your body requires, it turns to stored fat for energy. This balance is the key to losing weight.

How the Body Stores Excess Calories as Fat

When you eat more calories than your body can burn, the extra energy doesn't just disappear. Instead, your body converts these excess calories into fat, storing them for later use. This is your body's survival mechanism, designed to protect you during times of scarcity. In modern life, with easy access to high-calorie foods and less physical activity, we often take in more calories than we need, leading to fat accumulation over time.

Here's how it works: after digestion, the calories from your food are used for immediate energy needs, and any leftovers are converted into triglycerides, which are stored in fat cells. If this happens regularly, your fat stores increase, and you gain weight.

How the Body Uses Stored Fat for
Energy

On the flip side, when you create a calorie deficit by eating fewer calories than your body needs, your body starts to use its stored fat for energy. Essentially, your body breaks down the triglycerides stored in fat cells and converts them into energy that your muscles and organs can use. This process reduces the size of your fat cells, leading to weight loss.

Think of it as dipping into your savings account. When you're not taking in enough calories through food, your body taps into its fat reserves to make up the difference, fueling your daily activities. Over time, this is how fat loss occurs.

Why a Calorie Deficit Is Necessary for
Weight Loss

The concept of a *calorie deficit* is simple but powerful: you must burn more calories than you consume to lose weight. Without a calorie deficit, no matter how much you exercise or how healthy your food choices are, your body won't need to use its stored fat for energy, and weight loss won't occur.

This doesn't mean you need to starve yourself or drastically cut calories. A sustainable, moderate calorie deficit—about 500 to 1,000 fewer calories per day than your TDEE—can lead to safe and consistent weight loss of about 1 to 2 pounds per week. The key is balance: reducing your intake while still fueling your body with the nutrients it needs to feel energized and healthy.

In summary, calories matter in weight loss because they determine whether your body is in a state of fat storage or fat burning. By creating a calorie deficit, you encourage your body to use stored fat for energy, leading to gradual and sustainable weight loss.

Common Myths about Calories

When it comes to calories, there's no shortage of myths and misconceptions that can easily lead you astray on your weight loss journey. Let's clear up some of the most common myths about calories, so you can make more informed decisions about your health and nutrition.

The Myth of "Negative Calorie Foods"

One popular myth is that certain foods, like celery or grapefruit, are "negative calorie foods." The idea is that these foods require more energy to digest than the calories they provide, supposedly leading to weight loss simply by eating them.

While it's true that some foods are very low in calories—like leafy greens or cucumbers—the concept of negative calorie foods is misleading. Your body does use energy to digest food, known as the *Thermic Effect of Food* (TEF), but this usually accounts for only a small percentage of the calories consumed. Even with low-calorie foods, the amount of energy your body uses to digest them is not enough to create a calorie deficit. In short, no food can magically burn more calories than it contains. Weight loss always comes down to the balance between calories in and calories out.

Does All Fat Come from Excess Calories?

Another misconception is that all body fat comes directly from overeating or consuming excess calories. While a calorie surplus is the main cause of fat gain, the type of calories you consume—and how your body processes them—also plays a role.

For example, not all fats in the diet are stored as fat. Healthy fats, like those from avocados, nuts, and olive oil, are essential for bodily functions and don't necessarily contribute to fat gain when consumed in moderation. On the other hand, processed foods high in refined sugars and unhealthy fats can be more easily converted into stored fat, especially when they lead to overeating or spikes in insulin levels.

Moreover, your body's ability to store or burn fat can be influenced by factors like hormone levels, stress, and sleep patterns. So while excess calories are the main driver of fat gain, the bigger picture of health and lifestyle factors also matters.

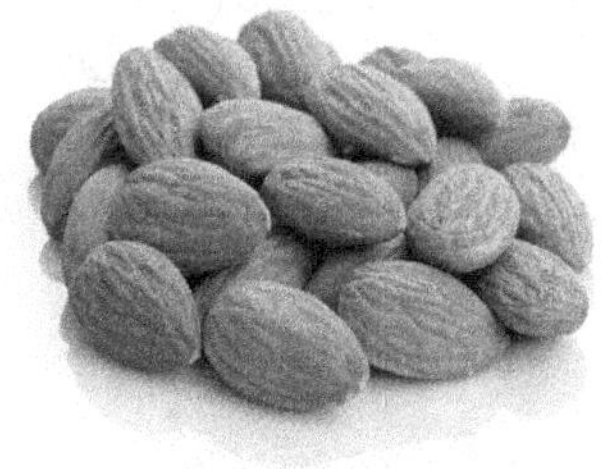

Why "Quality" of Calories Also Matters

One of the most persistent myths about calories is that "a calorie is just a calorie," implying that it doesn't matter where your calories come from as long as you stay within your limit. However, the *quality* of your calories is just as important as the quantity.

For example, 200 calories from a sugary snack like a candy bar will affect your body differently than 200 calories from a nutrient-dense source like a handful of almonds. The candy bar may give you a quick burst of energy, but it's likely to lead to a crash in blood sugar, leaving you hungry and craving more. Meanwhile, the almonds provide healthy fats, fiber, and protein that will keep you satisfied and energized for longer.

Nutrient-dense foods fuel your body with the vitamins, minerals, and macronutrients it needs to function at its best. They can help regulate your appetite, keep your metabolism running smoothly, and support overall health. In contrast, calorie-dense, nutrient-poor foods often leave you feeling hungry, leading to overeating and poor energy levels.

In summary, while calories are the foundation of weight management, the quality of those calories plays a significant role in your overall health, energy levels, and ability to stick to your goals. By focusing on nutrient-rich foods, you can make every calorie count toward a healthier, more sustainable lifestyle

Understanding Caloric Density and its Impact

One of the most effective tools for managing your weight and overall health is understanding *caloric density*—the number of calories a food contains relative to its weight or volume. Some foods pack a lot of calories into a small portion, while others offer fewer calories for a larger volume. Learning how to use caloric density to your advantage can help you make smarter food choices, stay satisfied, and control your calorie intake more easily.

Low vs. High-Calorie Density
Foods

Foods can be classified into two categories based on their caloric density:

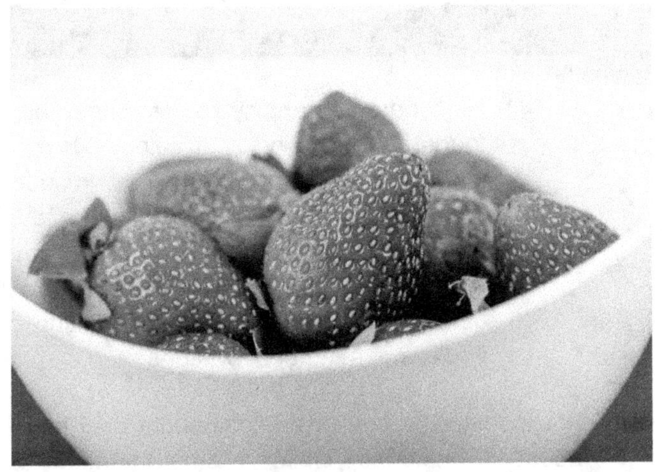

- **Low-calorie density foods**: These are foods that contain fewer calories per gram, meaning you can eat larger portions without consuming too many calories. Examples include fruits, vegetables, broth-based soups, and foods high in water or fiber.

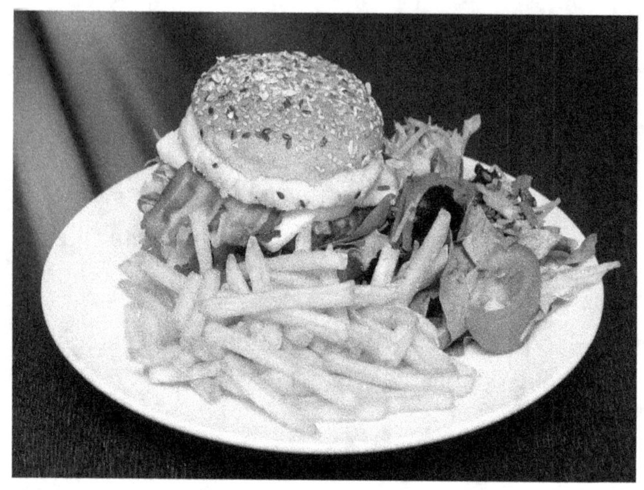

- **High-calorie density foods**: These are foods that pack a lot of calories into a smaller volume. Examples include processed snacks, fried foods, candy, oils, nuts, and full-fat dairy. While many high-calorie foods are tasty, they can quickly add up and lead to overeating if you're not mindful of portions.

For instance, a cup of broccoli might only have about 30 calories, while a small handful of almonds could have over 150 calories. You can eat much more of the low-calorie food and still take in fewer overall calories.

Caloric density plays a huge role in how full and satisfied you feel after eating. Low-calorie density foods, like vegetables, tend to be high in water and fiber, which fill you up without contributing a lot of calories. This means you can eat a larger volume of these foods and feel full without overloading on calories.

On the other hand, high-calorie density foods are often low in fiber and water, meaning they take up less space in your stomach and leave you feeling hungry sooner, despite consuming more calories. That's why you might polish off a bag of chips or a candy bar and still feel hungry, even though you've just eaten a significant number of calories.

By focusing on low-calorie density foods, you can eat more and feel fuller, while still maintaining a calorie deficit for weight loss.

Using Caloric Density to Plan
Meals

Planning meals with caloric density in mind is a simple but powerful strategy for weight management. You can make lower-calorie, nutrient-dense foods the foundation of your meals and snacks, allowing you to eat satisfying portions without exceeding your calorie goals.

Here's how to use caloric density to plan balanced meals:

1. **Start with low-calorie density foods**: Fill most of your plate with vegetables, fruits, and leafy greens. These foods provide bulk and nutrients with very few calories.
2. **Add moderate-calorie density foods**: Incorporate lean proteins like chicken, fish, tofu, or beans, as well as whole grains like brown rice or quinoa. These foods are more calorie-dense but provide essential nutrients and help keep you full.
3. **Be mindful with high-calorie density foods**: Use calorie-dense items like nuts, cheese, oils, and dressings in small amounts to enhance the flavor of your meals without going overboard on calories.

For example, a large salad filled with leafy greens, vegetables, a grilled chicken breast, a small portion of avocado, and a drizzle of olive oil creates a satisfying, nutrient-rich meal that keeps you full without being calorie-heavy.

By understanding and leveraging caloric density, you can design meals that are not only filling but also aligned with your weight management goals, making it easier to stay on track without feeling deprived.

Chapter 2: The Science of Weight Loss

What is metabolism?

Metabolism is often a buzzword in discussions about weight loss, and for good reason. It plays a crucial role in how your body uses energy and burns calories. Understanding what metabolism is, how it works, and the factors that influence it can give you a clearer picture of why some people lose weight more easily than others and how you can support your own weight loss efforts.

Definition of Metabolism

At its core, *metabolism* refers to all the chemical processes that occur in your body to keep you alive and functioning. These processes include breaking down food for energy, repairing cells, and maintaining body temperature. Your metabolism is essentially your body's engine, constantly working to convert the food you eat into energy that fuels everything you do, even when you're at rest.

Metabolism can be broken down into two main categories:

- **Basal Metabolic Rate (BMR)**: The number of calories your body needs to perform basic functions while at rest, such as breathing and maintaining your heart rate. Your BMR accounts for the majority of the calories you burn each day.
- **Active Metabolism**: The additional calories burned through physical activity and the digestion of food, also known as the *thermic effect of food (TEF)*. This includes everything from structured exercise to daily activities like walking or cleaning.

Factors that Influence Metabolism

Your metabolic rate is not fixed—it can be influenced by several factors, some of which are within your control, while others are not. Here are a few key factors that impact how fast or slow your metabolism runs:

1. **Age**: As you get older, your metabolism naturally slows down. This is partly due to a decrease in muscle mass and changes in hormones, making it harder to maintain the same level of calorie burn as when you were younger.

2. **Genetics**: Your genetic makeup plays a significant role in your metabolic rate. Some people are born with a naturally faster metabolism, while others have a slower one. While you can't change your genes, you can take steps to boost your metabolism through lifestyle choices.

3. **Muscle Mass**: Muscle tissue burns more calories than fat tissue, even at rest. This means that individuals with more muscle mass tend to have a higher BMR and burn more calories throughout the day. Strength training and building lean muscle can help increase your metabolic rate.

4. **Gender**: On average, men tend to have a higher metabolic rate than women because they generally have more muscle mass and larger body sizes. However, women can still optimize their metabolism through exercise and nutrition.

5. **Hormones**: Hormonal imbalances, such as those related to thyroid function, can affect your metabolism. For example, an underactive thyroid (hypothyroidism) can slow your metabolism, making weight loss more difficult, while an overactive thyroid (hyperthyroidism) can speed it up.

Metabolism plays a direct role in weight loss because it determines how many calories your body burns throughout the day. If your metabolism is slower, your body burns fewer calories, meaning you'll need to consume fewer calories or increase your activity level to create a calorie deficit and lose weight. Conversely, a faster metabolism allows you to burn more calories, making it easier to lose weight or maintain your current weight.

That said, while metabolism is important, it's not the only factor that influences weight loss. Even with a slower metabolism, you can still lose weight by focusing on creating a sustainable calorie deficit through a combination of diet and physical activity. Here are a few strategies to support a healthy metabolism:

- **Build muscle**: Strength training increases muscle mass, which boosts your BMR and helps you burn more calories, even when you're not exercising.
- **Stay active**: Regular physical activity, especially a mix of cardio and strength training, keeps your metabolism running efficiently and increases your daily calorie burn.

- **Eat enough protein**: Protein has a higher thermic effect than fats or carbohydrates, meaning your body uses more energy to digest it. Including protein-rich foods in your diet can help keep your metabolism elevated.
- **Get enough sleep**: Lack of sleep can disrupt hormones that regulate hunger and metabolism, making it harder to lose weight.

In summary, metabolism is a key player in weight loss, but it's not the whole story. While factors like age, genetics, and muscle mass influence your metabolic rate, you can still take control of your weight loss journey by focusing on lifestyle habits that support a healthy metabolism and create a sustainable calorie deficit

How to Boost Your Metabolism

While you may not have complete control over your metabolism, there are plenty of ways to give it a helpful nudge. By focusing on building muscle, making smart dietary choices, and adopting healthy lifestyle habits, you can increase your metabolic rate and make it easier to burn calories throughout the day. Let's dive into some practical ways to boost your metabolism.

One of the most effective ways to boost your metabolism is to build more muscle. Muscle tissue burns more calories than fat tissue, even when you're at rest, which means that having more muscle increases your Basal Metabolic Rate (BMR). The more muscle you have, the more calories your body burns, both during exercise and while at rest.

Strength training is the best way to increase muscle mass. Lifting weights or doing resistance exercises like bodyweight squats, lunges, push-ups, or using resistance bands can help you build lean muscle. When you engage in strength training, your body not only burns calories during the workout but also continues to burn calories afterward, a phenomenon known as *excess post-exercise oxygen consumption (EPOC)* or the "afterburn effect."

Incorporating strength training into your routine two to three times a week can have a lasting impact on your metabolism. Whether you use free weights, machines, or your own body weight, focusing on progressive overload (gradually increasing the weight or resistance) will help you build muscle and rev up your metabolism.

What you eat and how you fuel your body also has a significant impact on your metabolism. Certain dietary habits can help keep your metabolism running efficiently:

1. **Eat more protein**: Protein has a higher *thermic effect of food (TEF)* compared to carbohydrates and fats. This means your body uses more energy to digest and process protein, giving your metabolism a temporary boost after meals. Incorporating protein-rich foods like lean meats, fish, eggs, legumes, and nuts into your diet can help maintain muscle mass and keep your metabolism higher.

2. **Don't skip meals**: Skipping meals or eating too few calories can actually slow down your metabolism. When you don't eat enough, your body conserves energy by slowing its metabolic processes, making it harder to burn calories. Eating regular, balanced meals helps keep your metabolism running smoothly.

3. **Spice things up**: Some studies suggest that certain spices, like chili peppers, can slightly increase your metabolic rate. Capsaicin, the compound that

gives chili peppers their heat, may help you burn more calories after eating. While the effect is small, it doesn't hurt to add a little spice to your meals for an extra boost.

4. **Drink green tea or coffee**: Both green tea and coffee contain compounds that can temporarily increase metabolism. Green tea contains catechins, and coffee contains caffeine, both of which may boost calorie burning. Just be mindful of how much caffeine you consume, as too much can lead to jitters or sleep disruption.

Lifestyle Changes that Impact Metabolism

Beyond exercise and diet, certain lifestyle habits can also have a big influence on your metabolism. Making a few simple adjustments can help you keep your metabolic engine running efficiently:

1. **Get enough sleep**: Sleep is crucial for regulating hormones that affect metabolism. When you're sleep-deprived, hormones like leptin and ghrelin, which control hunger and satiety, become imbalanced. This can lead to increased cravings and a slower metabolism. Aim for 7 to 9 hours of

quality sleep each night to keep your metabolism on track.

2. **Stay hydrated**: Water is essential for your body's metabolic processes. Even mild dehydration can slow your metabolism, making it harder for your body to burn calories. Drinking water, especially cold water, may temporarily increase your metabolic rate as your body works to bring the water to body temperature. Aim to drink plenty of water throughout the day to stay hydrated and support metabolism.

3. **Manage stress**: Chronic stress can disrupt your metabolism by increasing levels of cortisol, a stress hormone that encourages the storage of fat, particularly around the belly. Finding ways to manage stress, whether through exercise, meditation, or relaxation techniques, can help keep your cortisol levels in check and support a healthy metabolism.

By focusing on building muscle, eating in ways that support metabolic health, and adopting healthy lifestyle habits like sleep, hydration, and stress management, you can give your metabolism the boost it needs. These changes may seem small, but over time, they can add up to a more efficient, calorie-burning body that supports your weight loss and health goals.

Metabolic rate myths

When it comes to metabolism, misinformation can often cloud judgment and lead to misguided dietary and lifestyle choices. To help you navigate the complexities of metabolism, let's debunk some common myths that can affect your understanding of how to effectively manage your weight and health.

Does Eating Small Meals Boost Metabolism?

One popular belief is that eating small, frequent meals throughout the day can boost your metabolism. While it's true that your body burns calories during the digestion process, known as the thermic effect of food (TEF), the difference in metabolic rate between eating small meals versus three larger meals is negligible.

In reality, the total number of calories you consume over the day is what matters most for weight management. Some studies suggest that meal frequency does not significantly impact metabolic rate or weight loss outcomes. What's more important is the overall quality and quantity of your food intake. Rather than obsessing over meal frequency, focus on finding a meal pattern that fits your lifestyle and keeps you feeling satisfied.

Another common myth is that certain foods can significantly "speed up" your metabolism. While some foods may have a slight thermogenic effect, the reality is that the impact is often minimal and not a magic solution for weight loss.

For instance, foods like chili peppers, green tea, and coffee contain compounds that can temporarily boost metabolic activity. However, the increase in calorie expenditure is usually modest and not enough to make a significant difference in weight loss on its own. The overall effect of these foods on your metabolism pales in comparison to the importance of total calorie intake and expenditure.

Additionally, relying solely on "metabolism-boosting" foods can lead to disappointment if they don't yield the results you expect. A balanced diet that includes a variety of nutrient-dense foods, combined with a healthy lifestyle, is far more effective for weight management than searching for a miracle food.

Many people wonder how much they can realistically change their metabolism through diet, exercise, or lifestyle modifications. While it's true that you can influence your metabolic rate, significant changes are often limited and take time.

Factors such as age, genetics, and hormonal balance are largely beyond your control and have a substantial impact on your metabolic rate. For example, as you age, your metabolism naturally slows down due to a decrease in muscle mass and changes in hormone levels.

When it comes to lifestyle interventions, such as strength training to build muscle, increasing muscle mass can lead to a higher BMR and more calories burned at rest. However, the increase may not be as dramatic as one might hope. Building a significant amount of muscle takes consistent effort and time, and while it can help raise your metabolic rate, the changes may be modest compared to your total calorie needs.

Ultimately, rather than focusing on how much your metabolism can change, it's more productive to concentrate on sustainable lifestyle habits that support your overall health and well-being. Remember, weight management is not just about boosting metabolism; it's about creating a balanced, healthy lifestyle that you can maintain long-term.

In summary, while there are many myths surrounding metabolism, understanding the facts can help you make informed choices about your health. Focus on what you can control—like diet quality, physical activity, and overall lifestyle—rather than chasing unrealistic expectations about metabolic changes. With the right approach, you can achieve your weight loss goals and improve your overall health.

How Weight Loss Happens

The Calorie Deficit Principle

Understanding the process of weight loss is crucial for anyone embarking on a journey to transform their body. At its core, weight loss occurs when you create a calorie deficit, meaning you burn more calories than you consume. However, several factors influence how this process unfolds, including metabolism, meal patterns, and food choices. Let's break down these elements to clarify how weight loss happens.

Does Eating Small Meals Boost Metabolism?

One common belief is that eating small, frequent meals throughout the day can enhance metabolism and lead to weight loss. While it's true that your body expends energy when digesting food (the thermic effect of food), research shows that meal frequency does not significantly impact your overall metabolic rate or weight loss.

In essence, whether you eat three larger meals or five to six smaller ones, the total caloric intake over the day is what matters most. The key is to find a meal pattern that fits your lifestyle and helps you feel satisfied without exceeding your calorie goals. Instead of fixating on meal frequency, focus on nutrient-dense foods that nourish your body while keeping your calorie intake in check.

Can Certain Foods "Speed Up" Metabolism?

Another prevalent myth is that certain foods can dramatically "speed up" metabolism and accelerate weight loss. While some foods may have a slight thermogenic effect (e.g., spicy foods like chili peppers, or drinks like green tea and coffee), the overall impact is often minimal.

The boost in metabolic rate from these foods is usually short-lived and not sufficient to account for substantial weight loss. Instead of seeking out "metabolism-boosting" foods as a quick fix, it's more effective to focus on a balanced diet that includes a variety of whole, nutrient-rich foods. This approach not only supports your metabolism but also provides the essential vitamins and minerals your body needs for overall health.

It's important to recognize that while you can influence your metabolic rate through lifestyle choices, significant changes may be limited. Factors such as age, genetics, and hormonal balance play a major role in determining your baseline metabolic rate. For instance, as you age, muscle mass typically decreases, leading to a natural decline in metabolism.

You can certainly take steps to increase your metabolic rate by building muscle through strength training. More muscle means a higher Basal Metabolic Rate (BMR), which translates to more calories burned at rest. However, the increase in metabolism from building muscle is usually modest and takes time and consistent effort.

Ultimately, weight loss is not solely about manipulating metabolism; it's about creating a sustainable calorie deficit through a combination of mindful eating and regular physical activity. Focus on incorporating healthy habits that support your goals—like strength training, eating nutrient-dense foods, and engaging in regular exercise—rather than chasing fleeting metabolic boosts.

Stages of weight loss

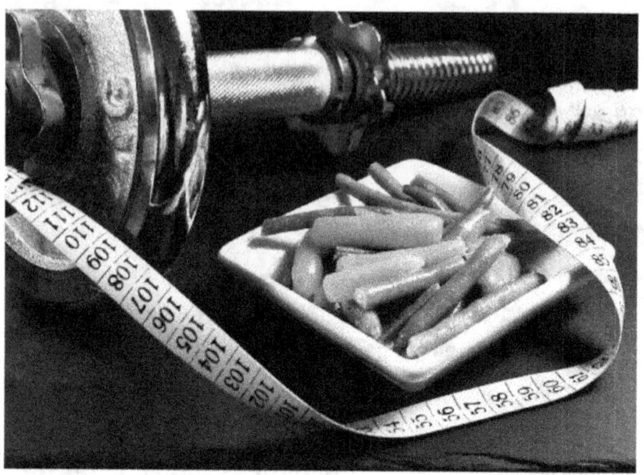

Weight loss is a multifaceted process that relies on creating a calorie deficit, and while metabolism plays a role, it's not the only factor. By understanding the myths and realities surrounding weight loss, you can make informed choices that align with your goals and lead to lasting results. Stay committed to a balanced lifestyle, and remember that sustainable changes will yield the best outcomes for your body and health.

Embarking on a weight loss journey can be both exciting and challenging. Understanding the different stages of weight loss can help you set realistic expectations and stay motivated as you work towards your goals. Each stage presents unique challenges and opportunities for growth. Let's explore the three main stages of weight loss: the early stage, the plateau stage, and long-term weight maintenance.

The Early Stage: Rapid Loss
Due to Water Weight

When you first start a weight loss program, it's common to experience rapid weight loss in the initial weeks. This initial drop is often attributed to the loss of water weight rather than fat. When you reduce your calorie intake or change your diet—especially if you lower your carbohydrate consumption—your body begins to deplete glycogen stores, which are the stored form of carbohydrates.

Glycogen binds to water in your body, so when glycogen is used for energy, the water is released. This can result in a significant decrease on the scale within the first few days or weeks. While this early stage can be encouraging, it's important to remember that this rapid loss is typically temporary and not a reflection of actual fat loss.

Understanding that this initial drop is mostly water weight can help you maintain a healthy perspective as you transition into the next stage of weight loss, where progress may become slower and more gradual.

After the initial phase, many individuals encounter what is often referred to as the "plateau stage." During this phase, weight loss may slow or even stall, leading to frustration and discouragement. This phenomenon occurs for several reasons:

1. **Metabolic Adaptation**: As you lose weight, your body's caloric needs decrease. With a lower body weight, your Basal Metabolic Rate (BMR) declines, meaning you burn fewer calories at rest. This can make it harder to maintain a calorie deficit, leading to slower weight loss.
2. **Muscle Loss**: Along with fat loss, some muscle mass may also be lost during a weight loss journey, especially if strength training is not part of the program. Since muscle tissue burns more calories than fat, losing muscle can further reduce your metabolic rate.
3. **Body's Regulatory Mechanisms**: Your body has natural regulatory mechanisms that promote energy balance. When you eat less and lose weight, your body may respond by increasing hunger hormones and decreasing hormones that signal

fullness, making you feel hungrier and more inclined to overeat.

To overcome a plateau, consider reassessing your caloric intake and physical activity levels. It may be beneficial to incorporate strength training to help preserve or rebuild muscle mass, as well as to make adjustments to your diet to ensure you are still in a calorie deficit.

Long-Term Weight Maintenance After Reaching Your Goal

Once you reach your weight loss goal, the journey doesn't end; maintaining that weight loss is often just as challenging as losing the weight in the first place. Successful long-term weight maintenance requires ongoing commitment and lifestyle changes.

Here are some strategies to help you maintain your weight loss:

1. **Continue Healthy Habits**: The habits that helped you lose weight—such as regular physical activity, mindful eating, and portion control—should continue to be part of your daily routine. These habits will not only help you maintain your weight but also contribute to overall health.

2. **Monitor Your Weight**: Regularly monitoring your weight can help you

stay aware of any changes and allow you to make adjustments as needed. Consider weighing yourself weekly or bi-weekly to catch any upward trends before they become significant.

3. **Set New Goals**: After achieving your initial weight loss goal, setting new fitness or health-related goals can keep you motivated. This could include running a race, mastering a new exercise, or exploring new healthy recipes.

4. **Be Flexible**: Life changes, and so will your weight. Accepting that fluctuations may occur can help you maintain a healthy mindset. Focus on the big picture and prioritize overall health rather than fixating on the scale.

5. **Seek Support**: Connecting with others who share similar goals can provide motivation and accountability. Whether it's friends, family, or a support group, having a network can make a significant difference in your long-term success.

In summary, weight loss is a journey with distinct stages, each with its own challenges and rewards. By understanding the early stage, the plateau stage, and the importance of long-term maintenance, you can better navigate your path and develop strategies to stay committed to your health and well-being. Remember, achieving and maintaining a healthy weight is a lifelong endeavor that requires patience, resilience, and a positive mindset.

The Role of Hormones in Weight Loss

Hormones play a crucial role in regulating various physiological processes in the body, including weight loss and management. Understanding how hormones like insulin, ghrelin, leptin, and cortisol influence your body can help you navigate your weight loss journey more effectively. Let's explore how these hormones impact fat storage, hunger, satiety, and overall weight loss.

How Insulin Impacts Fat Storage and Weight Loss

Insulin is a hormone produced by the pancreas that helps regulate blood sugar levels. When you eat carbohydrates, your body breaks them down into glucose (sugar), which enters the bloodstream. In response, insulin is released to facilitate the uptake of glucose into cells for energy or storage.

While insulin is essential for maintaining energy balance, its levels can significantly impact weight loss:

1. **Fat Storage**: Insulin promotes fat storage by encouraging the conversion

of excess glucose into fat in fat cells. When insulin levels are chronically high—often due to a diet high in refined carbohydrates and sugars—your body becomes less efficient at burning fat for energy, making weight loss more challenging.

2. **Inhibition of Fat Breakdown**: Elevated insulin levels can inhibit the breakdown of stored fat, making it difficult for your body to tap into its fat reserves. This means that if you are frequently consuming high-sugar or high-carb meals, you may be inadvertently promoting fat storage rather than fat loss.

To promote better insulin sensitivity and support weight loss, focus on eating a balanced diet that includes whole foods, fiber-rich fruits and vegetables, healthy fats, and lean proteins. These choices can help stabilize blood sugar levels and keep insulin responses in check.

Ghrelin and Leptin: Hormones that Control Hunger and Satiety

Ghrelin and leptin are two critical hormones that play opposing roles in hunger regulation:

1. **Ghrelin**: Often referred to as the "hunger hormone," ghrelin is produced in the stomach and signals hunger to

your brain. Levels of ghrelin increase when you are hungry and decrease after eating. When you're in a calorie deficit (eating fewer calories than your body needs), ghrelin levels may rise, increasing feelings of hunger and making it more difficult to stick to your weight loss plan.

2. **Leptin**: In contrast, leptin is produced by fat cells and signals satiety to the brain, helping to regulate energy balance. Higher levels of leptin are associated with increased feelings of fullness, while lower levels can lead to increased hunger. When you lose weight, your body's leptin levels decrease, which can lead to feelings of hunger and cravings, making it easy to regain weight.

The balance between ghrelin and leptin is crucial for effective weight management. To support healthy levels of these hormones, prioritize a balanced diet, regular physical activity, and adequate sleep. These lifestyle factors can help regulate hunger and satiety signals, making it easier to maintain a healthy weight.

*How Stress Hormones like
Cortisol Affect Fat Loss*

Cortisol, commonly known as the stress hormone, is produced by the adrenal glands in response to stress. While cortisol plays a necessary role in the body's stress response, chronic elevated levels can have negative effects on weight loss:

1. **Increased Appetite**: High levels of cortisol can lead to increased appetite and cravings, particularly for high-calorie, comfort foods. This can make it more challenging to adhere to a healthy eating plan.
2. **Fat Storage**: Elevated cortisol levels have been associated with increased fat storage, especially in the abdominal area. This type of fat, known as visceral fat, is linked to various health issues, including insulin resistance and metabolic syndrome.
3. **Muscle Breakdown**: Chronic stress and high cortisol levels can contribute to muscle breakdown, which can lower your metabolism. Maintaining muscle mass is essential for effective weight loss, as muscle tissue burns more calories at rest than fat tissue.

To manage cortisol levels and support weight loss, it's important to incorporate stress-reduction techniques into your daily routine. Activities such as mindfulness, yoga, regular exercise, and adequate sleep can help lower cortisol levels and promote a healthier hormonal balance.

Summary

Hormones play a vital role in the complex process of weight loss. Understanding how insulin impacts fat storage, how ghrelin and leptin regulate hunger and satiety, and the effects of stress hormones like cortisol can empower you to make informed choices that support your weight loss goals. By adopting a holistic approach that includes a balanced diet, regular physical activity, and stress management, you can create an environment conducive to effective weight management and overall health.

Chapter 3: Diet Strategies for Burning Calories

Types Of Diets And Their Effectiveness

Low-carb Diets (e.g., Keto, Atkins)

Low-carb diets, such as the Ketogenic (keto) and Atkins diets, have gained popularity for their effectiveness in promoting weight loss and improving metabolic health. These diets focus on significantly reducing carbohydrate intake, which influences how the body processes energy. Let's delve into how low-carb diets work, their benefits, and the challenges they may present.

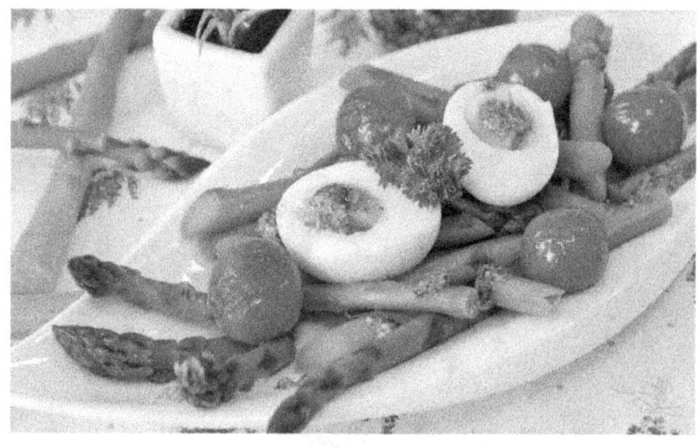

Low-carb diets operate on the principle of minimizing carbohydrate consumption, leading the body to rely on fat for energy instead of carbohydrates. Here's how this process unfolds:

- **Induction of Ketosis**: In a ketogenic diet, carbohydrate intake is typically reduced to a very low level (about 5-10% of total caloric intake), prompting the body to enter a state called ketosis. In this metabolic state, the liver converts fatty acids into ketones, which serve as an alternative energy source for the brain and body. This shift encourages the body to burn stored fat, facilitating weight loss.
- **Decreased Insulin Levels**: Lower carbohydrate intake results in reduced insulin production. Insulin is a hormone that promotes fat storage; with lower levels, the body is better equipped to utilize fat for energy. This helps prevent the accumulation of excess fat and promotes fat loss.
- **Enhanced Fat Oxidation**: As the body becomes more efficient at burning fat for fuel, individuals may experience a steady supply of energy, which can help reduce hunger and cravings. This can

make it easier to adhere to a calorie deficit, further supporting weight loss efforts.

Benefits: Rapid Fat Loss and Improved Metabolic Markers

Low-carb diets offer several compelling benefits, contributing to their effectiveness for weight loss and overall health:

- **Rapid Fat Loss**: One of the most appealing aspects of low-carb diets is the potential for rapid fat loss, especially in the initial stages. Many people experience a quick drop in weight due to the loss of water weight associated with reduced glycogen stores. This initial success can be motivating and encourage continued adherence to the diet.
- **Improved Metabolic Markers**: Research indicates that low-carb diets can lead to positive changes in metabolic health. These diets often result in reduced triglyceride levels, increased HDL (good) cholesterol, and improved blood sugar control. This can lower the risk of developing conditions such as type 2 diabetes and cardiovascular diseases.
- **Increased Satiety**: Low-carb diets tend to emphasize protein and healthy fats,

which can enhance feelings of fullness and satisfaction. This can help individuals manage their appetite more effectively, making it easier to stick to calorie goals without constant hunger.

Challenges: Sustainability and Potential Health Concerns

While low-carb diets can be effective, they come with challenges that may impact long-term adherence and overall health:

- **Sustainability**: Many individuals find it difficult to maintain a low-carb diet over time due to its restrictive nature. The elimination of many carbohydrate-rich foods can lead to feelings of deprivation and make social situations challenging. It's essential to create a plan that allows for some flexibility to increase the likelihood of long-term success.
- **Nutritional Deficiencies**: Severely limiting carbohydrates can result in nutritional deficiencies, particularly if whole food groups are excluded. Foods like fruits, whole grains, and legumes provide vital vitamins, minerals, and fiber, which are essential for optimal health. A well-rounded approach that includes a variety of nutrient-dense foods is crucial to avoid deficiencies.

- **Potential Health Concerns**: Some individuals may experience side effects when starting a low-carb diet, such as fatigue, digestive issues, or the so-called "keto flu" as the body adapts to ketosis. Additionally, a high intake of saturated fats—common in some low-carb diets—can raise concerns about cardiovascular health. It's important to focus on healthy fats, such as those found in avocados, nuts, seeds, and olive oil, while moderating saturated fat intake.

Summary

Low-carb diets, including ketogenic and Atkins approaches, can be effective tools for promoting weight loss and improving metabolic markers. By reducing carbohydrate intake, these diets encourage the body to burn fat for energy, leading to rapid fat loss and various health benefits. However, challenges related to sustainability and potential health concerns must be considered. As with any dietary approach, it's essential to find a plan that aligns with your lifestyle and health goals, ensuring long-term success and well-being. Always consider consulting with a healthcare professional or registered dietitian to personalize your approach and address any individual health concerns.

Intermittent Fasting

Intermittent fasting (IF) has gained significant popularity as a dietary approach for weight loss and overall health improvement. Unlike traditional diets that focus on what to eat, intermittent fasting emphasizes when to eat. By alternating between fasting and eating windows, individuals can manage their calorie Intake more effectively. Let's explore what intermittent fasting is, how it impacts calorie burning and fat loss, and some popular methods to consider.

What It Is: Fasting Windows and Eating Windows

Intermittent fasting involves cycling between periods of fasting (not eating) and eating. The key principle is to limit the time frame during which you consume food, allowing for extended periods without caloric intake. This approach can take several forms, but all variations share a common structure:

- **Fasting Windows**: During fasting windows, individuals abstain from calorie consumption. These periods can last anywhere from several hours to a full day, depending on the chosen method. Fasting can also encompass other non-caloric beverages, such as water, herbal tea, and black coffee.

- **Eating Windows**: In contrast, during eating windows, individuals consume their meals and snacks. The goal is to eat balanced meals that provide adequate nutrition while staying within caloric goals. The time allowed for eating can vary widely depending on the specific fasting protocol.

By creating structured eating patterns, intermittent fasting can help individuals become more mindful of their food choices and portion sizes.

How It Impacts Calorie Burning and Fat Loss

Intermittent fasting affects the body's metabolic processes in several ways that can promote fat loss:

- **Caloric Deficit**: By restricting the time frame for eating, intermittent fasting often leads to a natural reduction in calorie intake. Fewer hours in which to eat can make it easier to consume fewer calories overall, contributing to a calorie deficit—a fundamental requirement for weight loss.
- **Enhanced Fat Oxidation**: During fasting periods, the body depletes its glycogen stores and begins to rely on fat as its primary energy source. This shift

can enhance fat oxidation, promoting the utilization of stored fat for energy, especially during longer fasting periods.

- **Improved Insulin Sensitivity**: Intermittent fasting has been shown to improve insulin sensitivity, which can aid in better blood sugar regulation and fat storage management. Lower insulin levels during fasting can encourage fat loss and prevent fat accumulation.
- **Hormonal Changes**: Fasting triggers hormonal changes that facilitate fat burning. Levels of norepinephrine (a fat-burning hormone) increase during fasting, while growth hormone levels can also rise, promoting fat loss and muscle preservation.

Popular Methods: 16:8, 5:2, OMAD (One Meal a Day)

Several popular methods of intermittent fasting cater to different lifestyles and preferences. Here are three of the most widely adopted approaches:

- **16:8 Method**: This method involves fasting for 16 hours each day and restricting eating to an 8-hour window. For example, individuals may choose to eat between 12 PM and 8 PM, skipping breakfast but enjoying lunch and dinner. This approach is often considered one of the most manageable methods for beginners, as it fits well into many daily routines.

- **5:2 Diet**: In the 5:2 diet, individuals eat normally for five days of the week while restricting calorie intake to around 500-600 calories for two non-consecutive days. This method allows for flexibility, as individuals can choose which days to fast and what foods to consume on regular eating days.
- **OMAD (One Meal a Day)**: As the name suggests, the OMAD approach involves consuming just one meal per day, typically within a 1-hour eating window. While this method can lead to significant calorie restriction, it may require careful meal planning to ensure nutritional needs are met in a single sitting. OMAD can be more challenging for some people due to the extreme nature of the eating window.

Summary

Intermittent fasting presents a unique and flexible approach to weight management that emphasizes timing rather than specific food restrictions. By alternating between fasting and eating windows, individuals can create a calorie deficit, enhance fat burning, and improve metabolic health. However, it's essential to choose a method that fits your lifestyle and ensures balanced nutrition. As with any dietary change, consider consulting with a healthcare professional or registered dietitian to determine the best approach for your individual needs and goals. With the right plan, intermittent fasting can be a powerful tool for achieving lasting weight loss and overall well-being.

Calorie Counting and Flexible Dieting

Calorie counting and flexible dieting are powerful strategies for individuals looking to manage their weight while still enjoying their favorite foods. By tracking calorie intake and balancing macronutrients, you can create a sustainable eating pattern that supports your health and weight loss goals. Let's explore the essentials of calorie counting, how to balance macronutrients, and the importance of flexibility to prevent diet burnout.

Tracking Your Intake: Apps and Methods

One of the foundational principles of calorie counting is tracking your food intake. Fortunately, technology has made this process easier and more accessible than ever. Here are some popular methods and tools:

- **Mobile Apps**: Numerous smartphone apps, such as MyFitnessPal, Lose It!, and Cronometer, allow users to log their food intake effortlessly. These apps often come with extensive databases of foods and their calorie counts, making it simple to track meals and snacks accurately. Many also provide features for scanning barcodes and creating custom recipes, which can enhance usability.

- **Food Diaries**: If you prefer a more hands-on approach, maintaining a food diary can be an effective way to track your intake. Writing down everything you eat, including portion sizes, can help you stay accountable and provide insight into your eating patterns. This method also encourages mindfulness about food choices.
- **Measuring Tools**: Utilizing kitchen scales and measuring cups can help you gain a better understanding of portion sizes. While it may seem tedious at first, measuring your food can improve your accuracy in calorie counting and help you develop a more intuitive sense of serving sizes over time.

Calorie counting isn't just about keeping track of numbers; it's also about understanding the composition of your diet. Balancing macronutrients—proteins, fats, and carbohydrates—is crucial for achieving your nutritional goals and supporting overall health. Here's a breakdown of each macronutrient:

- **Proteins**: Essential for building and repairing tissues, proteins also play a vital role in satiety. Incorporating lean protein sources such as chicken, fish, beans, and legumes into your meals can help you feel fuller for longer, making it easier to stick to your calorie goals.
- **Fats**: Healthy fats, like those found in avocados, nuts, seeds, and olive oil, are vital for hormone production and overall health. They also contribute to feelings of fullness, helping to curb cravings. Aim for a balance of monounsaturated, polyunsaturated, and saturated fats while keeping overall fat intake within a reasonable range.
- **Carbohydrates**: Carbs are the body's primary source of energy, particularly for high-intensity activities. Choose whole, minimally processed carbohydrate sources, such as whole grains, fruits,

and vegetables. These foods are rich in nutrients and fiber, which can support digestive health and help maintain steady energy levels.

To determine your ideal macronutrient ratios, consider factors such as your activity level, weight loss goals, and personal preferences. Finding a balance that works for you can enhance your overall experience with calorie counting.

Allowing Flexibility to Avoid Diet Burnout

One of the most significant benefits of flexible dieting is its emphasis on balance and moderation. Allowing yourself some flexibility in your diet can help prevent feelings of deprivation and, ultimately, diet burnout. Here's how to incorporate flexibility into your calorie counting routine:

- **Incorporate Treats**: Rather than completely eliminating your favorite foods, incorporate them into your calorie budget. Whether it's a slice of pizza or a piece of chocolate, allowing yourself to enjoy treats in moderation can satisfy cravings and make your diet more enjoyable.
- **Focus on Quality**: While tracking calories is essential, it's equally

important to consider the quality of the foods you consume. Prioritize nutrient-dense foods that provide essential vitamins and minerals, while still allowing for occasional indulgences. This approach fosters a healthy relationship with food and prevents the all-or-nothing mentality.

- **Adjust Your Approach**: Life is dynamic, and your dietary needs may change based on factors like physical activity, stress levels, and social events. Be willing to adjust your calorie intake and macronutrient balance as needed. This adaptability can lead to a more sustainable approach to dieting and long-term weight management.

Summary

Calorie counting and flexible dieting offer effective strategies for managing weight while maintaining a balanced and enjoyable relationship with food. By tracking your intake using apps or food diaries, balancing macronutrients, and allowing for flexibility, you can create a sustainable dietary approach that supports your health and weight loss goals. Remember, the key to success lies in finding a balance that works for you, so you can enjoy the journey to better health without feeling deprived. With a mindful approach to eating, you can achieve lasting results and enjoy a high-quality life while transforming your body.

PRACTICAL TIPS FOR SUSTAINABLE CALORIC REDUCTION

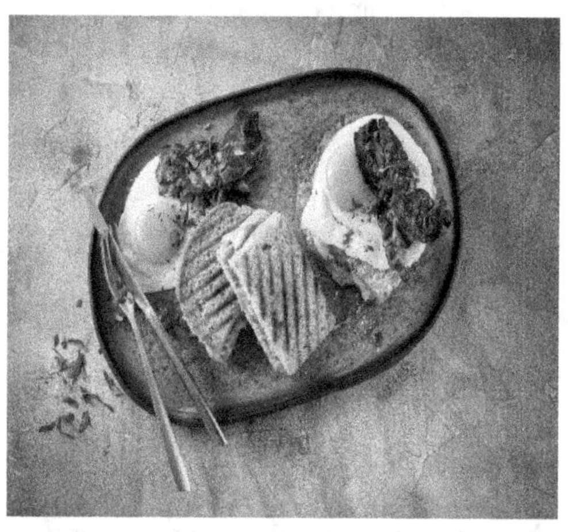

Reducing Portion Sizes

Reducing portion sizes is a practical and effective strategy for achieving sustainable caloric reduction and managing weight. By being mindful of how much food you consume, you can create a calorie deficit without feeling deprived. Here are some practical tips to help you control portions, feel satisfied with smaller meals, and use visual cues to aid in portion control.

- **Measure and Weigh**: Start by measuring and weighing your food, especially for high-calorie items like nuts, oils, or grains. Using a food scale can help you become more aware of portion sizes and ensure you are not unintentionally overeating. Gradually, you'll develop a better intuition for appropriate serving sizes.

- **Serve Smaller Portions**: When serving food, dish out smaller portions to begin with. You can always go back for seconds if you're still hungry, but starting with a smaller plateful can help reduce the likelihood of overeating.

- **Mindful Eating**: Practice mindful eating by slowing down and savoring each bite. Focus on the flavors, textures, and aromas of your food. This practice can enhance your eating experience and help you recognize when you're satisfied, reducing the chances of consuming larger portions.

How to "Feel Full" with Smaller Meals

- **Incorporate Fiber**: Foods high in fiber, such as fruits, vegetables, legumes, and whole grains, can help you feel fuller with fewer calories. Fiber adds bulk to your meals, promoting satiety and slowing digestion. Aim to fill half your plate with non-starchy vegetables to maximize volume while minimizing calories.

- **Choose Protein-Rich Foods**: Protein has a high satiety value, meaning it can help you feel full longer. Include lean sources of protein, like chicken, fish, eggs, or plant-based options like tofu and beans, in your meals. Pairing protein with fiber-rich foods can enhance feelings of fullness.

- **Stay Hydrated**: Sometimes, thirst is mistaken for hunger. Drink water before and during meals to help control hunger cues. Including hydrating foods, such as fruits and soups, can also contribute to your overall fluid intake and help you feel satisfied with smaller meals.

Using Plate Size and Visual Cues to Control Portions

- **Choose Smaller Plates and Bowls**: The size of your dinnerware can significantly influence portion sizes. Opt for smaller plates, bowls, and utensils to create the illusion of a fuller plate. Studies show that using smaller dishes can lead to reduced food intake while still satisfying your visual cues for a full meal.

- **Visual Cues**: Familiarize yourself with visual cues for appropriate portion sizes. For example, a serving of protein should be about the size of your palm, while a serving of carbohydrates can be roughly the size of your fist. Use these visual markers to guide your portion sizes when eating.
- **Divide Your Plate**: Consider using the "plate method" to visually allocate space for different food groups. Fill half your plate with vegetables, one-quarter with protein, and one-quarter with whole grains or starchy foods. This method not only promotes portion control but also ensures you're getting a balanced meal.

Summary

Reducing portion sizes is a simple yet effective strategy for achieving sustainable caloric reduction and supporting weight management. By implementing practical tips for portion control, focusing on high-fiber and protein-rich foods to enhance feelings of fullness, and using visual cues to guide portion sizes, you can create a satisfying eating experience without feeling deprived. Remember, sustainable weight loss is about making manageable changes that fit into your lifestyle. With a mindful approach to portion sizes, you can enjoy your meals while working toward your health and fitness goals.

Healthy Food Swaps

Making healthy food swaps is an effective strategy for reducing calorie intake without sacrificing flavor or satisfaction. By replacing high-calorie foods with lower-calorie alternatives and adopting healthier cooking methods, you can create meals that are both nutritious and delicious. Here's a guide to help you identify beneficial food swaps, cooking methods that lower calorie content, and nutrient-dense, low-calorie foods.

Swapping High-Calorie Foods
for Lower-Calorie Alternatives

- **Dairy Alternatives**: Replace full-fat dairy products with lower-calorie versions. For example, choose Greek yogurt or cottage cheese instead of sour cream or cream cheese. Opt for skim or almond milk instead of whole milk in your coffee or cereal. These swaps can significantly reduce calories while still providing essential nutrients.
- **Condiments and Sauces**: Many condiments can be calorie traps. Swap mayonnaise for mustard or hummus, which are typically lower in calories and higher in flavor. Similarly, choose salsa

or vinegar-based dressings over creamy dressings to add taste without excess calories.

- **Snacks**: Instead of reaching for chips or cookies, opt for air-popped popcorn, veggie sticks with salsa, or a small handful of nuts. These alternatives provide crunch and satisfaction without the added calories of traditional snack foods.
- **Carbohydrate Swaps**: For a lower-calorie carbohydrate option, replace white rice with cauliflower rice or quinoa. Instead of traditional pasta, try spiralized zucchini (zoodles) or whole-grain pasta to increase fiber and nutrients while reducing calories.

Cooking Methods that Reduce Calorie Content

- **Grilling vs. Frying**: Grilling, baking, or steaming foods can significantly reduce calorie content compared to frying. Frying often requires additional oil, which adds extra calories. Grilled chicken, fish, or vegetables can achieve a delicious flavor without the added fat.
- **Broiling**: Broiling is another great cooking method that uses high heat from above to cook food quickly, resulting in less fat absorption compared

to frying. It's an excellent option for cooking meats and vegetables while keeping calorie counts low.

- **Roasting**: Roasting vegetables with minimal olive oil or seasoning can enhance their natural flavors without the need for calorie-dense sauces. Roasted veggies like Brussels sprouts, carrots, and sweet potatoes can be satisfying and nutritious side dishes.
- **Using Non-Stick Cookware**: Investing in non-stick pans can help reduce the need for oil when cooking. This simple change allows you to prepare eggs, stir-fries, and more with less added fat, contributing to lower calorie meals.

Choosing Nutrient-Dense, Low-Calorie Foods

- **Fruits and Vegetables**: Load your plate with colorful fruits and vegetables, which are typically low in calories and high in essential vitamins and minerals. Foods like berries, leafy greens, cucumbers, and bell peppers are excellent choices that can fill you up without adding many calories.
- **Lean Proteins**: Incorporate lean protein sources such as skinless chicken, turkey, fish, and legumes. These options provide the protein necessary for

muscle maintenance and satiety while being lower in calories compared to fatty cuts of meat.

- **Whole Grains**: Opt for whole grains like brown rice, quinoa, or oats instead of refined grains. Whole grains are more nutrient-dense and provide fiber, which can help you feel fuller for longer, making them a smart choice for those looking to manage their weight.
- **Legumes and Pulses**: Beans, lentils, and chickpeas are fantastic nutrient-dense foods that are high in fiber and protein. They can be used as meat substitutes in many dishes, providing a satisfying texture and taste while being lower in calories.

Summary

Healthy food swaps can significantly impact your caloric intake while still allowing you to enjoy delicious meals. By swapping high-calorie foods for lower-calorie alternatives, employing cooking methods that reduce calorie content, and choosing nutrient-dense, low-calorie foods, you can create a balanced diet that supports your weight loss goals. These small changes can lead to sustainable habits and a healthier lifestyle, empowering you to enjoy food while making progress toward your health and wellness objectives.

Eating Mindfully to Reduce Caloric Intake

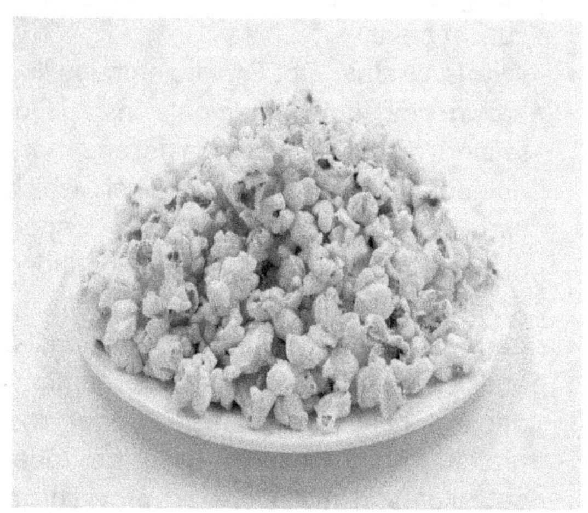

Mindful eating is a powerful practice that can help you become more aware of your food choices and consumption habits, ultimately leading to reduced caloric intake and improved health. By slowing down, recognizing emotional triggers, and planning your meals, you can cultivate a more mindful approach to eating. Here are key strategies to help you eat mindfully and effectively manage your caloric intake.

Slowing Down while Eating to Recognize Fullness

- **Savor Each Bite**: Take the time to truly savor your food. Focus on the flavors, textures, and aromas of each bite. Chewing slowly and thoroughly not only enhances your eating experience but also allows your brain to register fullness signals more effectively.

- **Put Down Your Utensils**: After each bite, set down your fork or spoon. This simple action encourages you to pause and gives your body time to signal when it's satisfied. By creating this space, you can become more in tune with your hunger cues and prevent overeating.
- **Eliminate Distractions**: Eating while distracted—whether by screens, books, or conversations—can lead to mindless eating and overconsumption. Try to eat in a calm environment, focusing solely on your meal. This practice can help you recognize your body's signals and enjoy your food more fully.

Avoiding Emotional Eating
Triggers

- **Identify Your Triggers**: Take a moment to reflect on your eating habits and identify situations or emotions that prompt you to eat when you're not hungry. Whether it's stress, boredom, or loneliness, recognizing these triggers is the first step toward managing them.
- **Find Alternative Coping Strategies**: Instead of turning to food during emotional moments, develop alternative

coping strategies. Consider activities like going for a walk, practicing deep breathing, journaling, or engaging in a hobby to help manage stress or boredom without involving food.

- **Practice Mindfulness Techniques**: Incorporate mindfulness practices such as meditation or yoga into your routine. These techniques can help you cultivate a deeper awareness of your thoughts and emotions, reducing the likelihood of emotional eating and promoting healthier choices.

Planning Meals to Prevent Overeating

- **Meal Prep**: Take time to plan and prepare your meals in advance. Having pre-portioned, healthy meals ready to go can help you resist the temptation to indulge in high-calorie, convenience foods when hunger strikes. Meal prepping allows you to control portions and ingredients, making it easier to stay on track with your goals.
- **Create a Balanced Plate**: When planning meals, aim to create balanced plates that include a variety of food groups—lean protein, healthy fats, whole grains, and plenty of fruits and vegetables. This balance can help

ensure that you're getting adequate nutrition while also promoting satiety.

- **Mindful Snacking**: Plan your snacks just as you would your meals. Choose nutrient-dense options that are high in fiber and protein, such as fruit with nut butter, yogurt with berries, or raw veggies with hummus. Having healthy snacks on hand can help prevent impulsive eating and keep your energy levels steady throughout the day.

Summary

Eating mindfully is a valuable approach to reducing caloric intake while enhancing your overall relationship with food. By slowing down during meals, recognizing and managing emotional eating triggers, and planning your meals in advance, you can foster a more conscious eating experience that aligns with your health goals. Mindful eating not only supports weight management but also cultivates a deeper appreciation for the food you enjoy, ultimately leading to a healthier, more fulfilling lifestyle.

Chapter 4: Exercise and Activity to Burn More Calories

Types Of Exercises For Maximum Calorie Burn

Cardiovascular Exercises

Cardiovascular exercises, often referred to as cardio, are an essential component of any fitness routine aimed at maximizing calorie burn and promoting fat loss. These activities elevate your heart rate, improve lung capacity, and boost overall endurance. Here's a closer look at popular cardiovascular exercises, how they increase calorie burn, and the best options for fat loss.

Examples: Running, Cycling, Swimming

- **Running**: One of the most effective forms of cardio, running can be done outdoors or on a treadmill. It's accessible and requires minimal equipment—just a good pair of running shoes. Whether you're jogging at a steady pace or engaging in interval sprints, running can burn a significant number of calories.

- **Cycling**: Whether you choose to cycle outdoors on a road or trail or participate in stationary biking classes, cycling is a fantastic low-impact cardio exercise. It's great for building leg strength while providing an excellent cardiovascular workout. The intensity can be adjusted based on speed and resistance.
- **Swimming**: Swimming is a full-body workout that engages multiple muscle groups while being easy on the joints. It's an effective way to improve cardiovascular fitness and endurance. Different strokes—such as freestyle, breaststroke, or butterfly—can vary the intensity and calorie burn.

How they Increase your Calorie Burn

- **Elevated Heart Rate**: Cardiovascular exercises elevate your heart rate, which increases blood circulation and oxygen delivery to muscles. As your heart works harder, your body burns more calories. The higher the intensity of the exercise, the more calories you'll burn per minute.
- **Duration and Intensity**: The number of calories burned during cardio is influenced by both the duration and intensity of the workout. Longer sessions at moderate intensity or

shorter, high-intensity interval training (HIIT) workouts can effectively boost calorie expenditure. Both approaches have their benefits, and mixing them into your routine can optimize results.

- **Afterburn Effect**: Engaging in high-intensity cardio can lead to excess post-exercise oxygen consumption (EPOC), commonly referred to as the "afterburn" effect. After intense workouts, your body continues to burn calories at an elevated rate as it recovers, contributing to additional calorie burn beyond the exercise session itself.

Best Cardio Exercises for Fat Loss

- **High-Intensity Interval Training (HIIT)**: This workout method alternates between short bursts of intense exercise and brief recovery periods. HIIT has been shown to burn a high number of calories in a short time while promoting fat loss and improving metabolic function.
- **Circuit Training**: Combining cardio and strength exercises in a circuit can effectively elevate your heart rate while building muscle. By alternating between exercises with minimal rest, you can

maintain a high calorie burn throughout the workout.

- **Group Classes**: Participating in group fitness classes such as spin, Zumba, or kickboxing can make cardio fun and engaging. The camaraderie and motivation of a group setting often encourage participants to push harder, leading to greater calorie burn.
- **Rowing**: Using a rowing machine is an excellent full-body workout that engages both upper and lower body muscles. It can be an effective form of cardio for fat loss, providing both aerobic benefits and muscle strengthening.

Summary

Incorporating cardiovascular exercises into your fitness routine is vital for maximizing calorie burn and promoting fat loss. Activities like running, cycling, and swimming offer diverse options that can suit different preferences and fitness levels. By understanding how these exercises increase calorie burn and choosing the most effective forms of cardio for your goals, you can create a balanced workout plan that supports your weight loss journey while improving overall health and fitness.

Strength Training

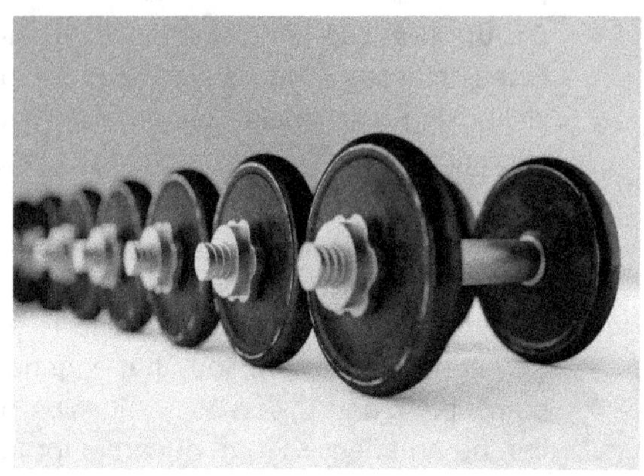

Strength training is not just for those looking to bulk up; it's a fundamental practice for anyone aiming to maximize calorie burn, enhance fat loss, and achieve a toned physique. By incorporating strength training into your fitness routine, you can build muscle, increase your resting metabolic rate, and reshape your body. Let's explore the key aspects of strength training and its effectiveness in your weight loss journey.

*Building Muscle to Increase
Resting Metabolic Rate*

- **Muscle Mass Matters**: Muscle tissue is metabolically active, meaning it requires more energy (calories) to maintain than fat tissue does. This translates into a higher resting metabolic rate (RMR) for individuals with greater muscle mass.

Essentially, the more muscle you have, the more calories you burn at rest.

- **Caloric Burn Over Time**: Research indicates that gaining even a small amount of muscle can lead to a noticeable increase in daily caloric burn. For example, adding just 2-3 pounds of muscle can boost your RMR by about 10-30 calories a day. While this might not seem significant at first glance, over weeks and months, these additional calories can add up, aiding in weight management.

- **Afterburn Effect**: Strength training also promotes a prolonged calorie burn due to the recovery process. After your workout, your body continues to burn calories as it repairs muscle fibers and restores energy levels, a phenomenon known as excess post-exercise oxygen consumption (EPOC). This effect can last several hours post-workout, contributing to your overall daily calorie expenditure.

*Compound vs. Isolation
Exercises for Weight Loss*

- **Compound Exercises**: These exercises engage multiple muscle groups simultaneously, making them highly efficient for calorie burning and overall strength development. Examples include squats, deadlifts, bench presses, and rows. Because compound exercises require more energy and coordination, they tend to burn more calories both during and after the workout.

- **Isolation Exercises**: In contrast, isolation exercises target a specific muscle group and involve movement at a single joint. Examples include bicep curls, tricep extensions, and leg curls. While these exercises can help you build muscle definition and improve strength in specific areas, they generally do not yield the same level of calorie burn as compound movements.
- **Balanced Approach**: A comprehensive strength training program often combines both compound and isolation exercises. This balance allows you to enhance overall muscle growth, improve strength, and achieve a well-rounded physique. While compound exercises can help with overall fat loss, isolation exercises can fine-tune specific muscles and improve muscle symmetry.

- **Fat Loss**: Strength training is an effective strategy for fat loss. By creating a calorie deficit—burning more calories than you consume—strength training helps your body utilize stored fat for energy. The combination of building muscle and losing fat leads to a healthier body composition and a leaner appearance.

- **Muscle Toning**: The term "toning" often refers to the process of reducing body fat while developing muscle definition. Strength training enhances muscle definition and makes it more visible. By focusing on building muscle through resistance training and maintaining a healthy diet, you can achieve a sculpted, toned look.

- **Functional Benefits**: Beyond aesthetics, strength training improves functional strength, making everyday activities easier. Increased muscle strength enhances your ability to perform daily tasks, reduces the risk of injury, and supports your overall fitness goals. Moreover, a stronger body can improve your performance in other exercises, including cardio workouts.

Summary

Strength training is a crucial aspect of any weight loss program, helping to maximize calorie burn, promote fat loss, and enhance muscle tone. By understanding how building muscle increases your resting metabolic rate, recognizing the differences between compound and isolation exercises, and acknowledging the benefits of strength training for fat loss, you can develop a well-rounded fitness routine that aligns with your goals. Embrace strength training as a powerful tool in your weight loss journey, and watch as it transforms your body and boosts your overall health.

High-Intensity Interval Training (HIIT)

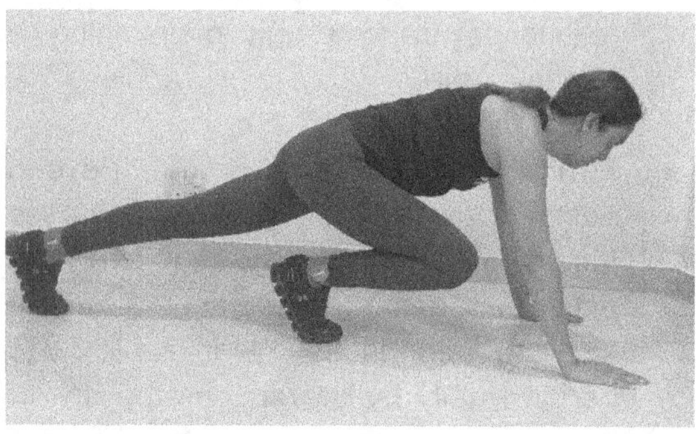

High-Intensity Interval Training (HIIT) has gained popularity in the fitness world for its ability to burn calories quickly and efficiently. This form of exercise alternates between short bursts of intense activity and brief recovery periods, making it an excellent choice for those looking to maximize their workout in a limited amount of time. Let's explore how HIIT burns calories, the benefits of afterburn, and some example workouts for different fitness levels.

How HIIT Burns Calories
Quickly and Efficiently

- **Maximal Effort**: HIIT is characterized by short, intense bouts of exercise that push you to your limits, followed by periods of rest or lower-intensity activity. This approach maximizes calorie burn in a short amount of time, often more effectively than traditional steady-state cardio workouts. In just 20-30 minutes of HIIT, you can burn as many calories as you would in an hour of moderate exercise.
- **Increased Heart Rate**: The intensity of HIIT elevates your heart rate rapidly, leading to increased caloric expenditure. Because you're working at a higher intensity, your body demands more energy, resulting in greater calorie burn during the workout.
- **Time-Efficient**: HIIT workouts can be completed in a fraction of the time compared to traditional cardio sessions. This makes HIIT an attractive option for

those with busy schedules who still want an effective workout. You can fit in a HIIT session in as little as 15-30 minutes, making it easier to incorporate into your daily routine.

Benefits of Afterburn (Excess Post-Exercise Oxygen Consumption)

- **What is Afterburn?**: After a HIIT workout, your body enters a recovery phase known as Excess Post-Exercise Oxygen Consumption (EPOC). During this time, your body continues to burn calories at an elevated rate as it restores itself to pre-exercise levels. This process includes repairing muscle tissues, replenishing energy stores, and returning your heart rate to baseline levels.
- **Caloric Burn Beyond the Workout**: The afterburn effect can lead to additional calorie burn for hours or even days post-exercise. Research suggests that HIIT can increase your metabolic rate for up to 24-48 hours after your workout. This means that the benefits of your HIIT session extend beyond the workout itself, contributing to weight loss and improved fitness.

- **Improved Metabolism**: The combination of intense exercise and the afterburn effect can enhance your metabolism, making your body more efficient at burning calories throughout the day. This can be especially beneficial for those looking to lose weight or maintain a healthy weight over time.

Types of HIIT Workouts

- **Beginner HIIT Workout:**
  Warm-up: 5 minutes of light cardio (e.g., brisk walking or cycling).
  Workout: Repeat the following circuit 3 times, resting for 1 minute between rounds:
    - 30 seconds of bodyweight squats
    - 30 seconds of push-ups (knee push-ups for beginners)
    - 30 seconds of jumping jacks
    - 30 seconds of rest
  Cool Down: 5 minutes of stretching.
- **Intermediate HIIT Workout:**
  Warm-up: 5 minutes of dynamic stretching or light cardio.
  Workout: Repeat the following circuit 4 times, resting for 30 seconds between rounds:
    - 40 seconds of burpees

- 40 seconds of mountain climbers
- 40 seconds of kettlebell swings (or dumbbell swings)
- 40 seconds of high knees
- 40 seconds of rest

Cool Down: 5-10 minutes of stretching to promote recovery.

Summary

High-Intensity Interval Training (HIIT) is an incredibly effective way to burn calories quickly and efficiently, making it a valuable tool in your weight loss journey. With the added benefits of afterburn, which boosts calorie burn even after your workout is done, HIIT can significantly contribute to your overall fitness and weight management goals. By incorporating HIIT into your exercise routine, you can achieve a high level of intensity in a shorter time frame, making it easier to stay consistent and motivated on your path to a healthier lifestyle.

INCREASING DAILY ACTIVITY

Non-Exercise Activity Thermogenesis (NEAT)

When it comes to weight management, most people focus on structured exercise routines, often overlooking the significant impact of daily non-exercise activities on calorie burn. This is where Non-Exercise Activity Thermogenesis (NEAT) comes into play. NEAT encompasses all the calories you burn through activities that are not deliberate exercise, such as walking, fidgeting, or even standing. Let's dive into what NEAT is, how it impacts calorie burn, and simple ways to increase your daily activity.

What is NEAT and How It Impacts Calorie Burn

- **Understanding NEAT**: NEAT refers to the energy expended for everything we do that is not sleeping, eating, or engaging in formal exercise. This includes activities like walking to your car, gardening, cleaning, and even fidgeting while sitting. While individual NEAT contributions may seem small, they can add up significantly throughout the day.
- **Caloric Contribution**: Research has shown that NEAT can account for a substantial portion of daily calorie expenditure. Depending on lifestyle and activity levels, NEAT can contribute anywhere from 15% to 50% of total daily energy expenditure (TDEE). For example, a person with a sedentary job who engages in minimal movement may

burn fewer calories compared to someone with an active job who regularly moves around throughout the day.

- **Impact on Weight Loss**: Because NEAT can vary widely between individuals, it plays a crucial role in weight management. Some people naturally have higher NEAT levels and, as a result, may find it easier to maintain a healthy weight. Conversely, those who are more sedentary may struggle with weight gain, even if they exercise regularly.

Simple Ways to Increase NEAT: Walking, Fidgeting, Standing

- **Incorporate More Walking**: One of the simplest ways to increase NEAT is to walk more. Consider parking further away from entrances, taking the stairs instead of the elevator, or going for short walks during breaks. Aim for 10-15 minutes of walking throughout your day; these short bursts can significantly boost your overall activity level.
- **Fidgeting Counts**: Even small movements like tapping your feet, drumming your fingers, or shifting in your chair can contribute to NEAT. While these actions may seem minor,

they add up over time and can increase your daily caloric burn.

- **Opt for Standing or Active Options**: If possible, consider using a standing desk or taking phone calls while standing. You can also incorporate movement into your day by doing household chores, gardening, or engaging in activities that require you to be on your feet. Even simple changes like pacing while talking or stretching can make a difference.

How NEAT Can Contribute to Long-Term Fat Loss

- **Sustainable Lifestyle Changes**: Increasing NEAT is an effective way to promote long-term fat loss because it encourages a more active lifestyle without the need for structured exercise programs. Small, consistent changes can lead to significant results over time, making it easier to integrate activity into your daily routine.
- **Cumulative Effects**: When combined with regular exercise, higher levels of NEAT can create a larger calorie deficit, supporting weight loss goals. The key is to find enjoyable activities that seamlessly fit into your life, making it sustainable in the long run.

- **Preventing Weight Regain**: Studies indicate that maintaining higher levels of NEAT can help prevent weight regain after initial weight loss. By staying active throughout the day, you increase your overall energy expenditure, which can be crucial for maintaining a healthy weight.

Summary

Non-Exercise Activity Thermogenesis (NEAT) is a powerful tool for increasing calorie burn and supporting weight loss without requiring structured exercise. By understanding what NEAT is and how it impacts daily calorie expenditure, you can identify simple, effective ways to boost your activity levels. Incorporating more walking, fidgeting, and standing into your routine can contribute to long-term fat loss and help you create a sustainable, active lifestyle. Remember, every little bit counts—small changes can lead to big results over time.

Creating a Daily Activity Routine

Establishing a daily activity routine is essential for maintaining a healthy lifestyle and achieving weight loss goals. By incorporating regular movement into your day-to-day activities, you can boost your calorie burn, enhance your overall well-being, and create sustainable habits that last a lifetime. Here, we'll explore how to create an effective daily activity routine that includes walking, movement at work, and staying active outside of the gym.

- **Daily Step Goal**: A common benchmark for daily physical activity is to aim for 10,000 steps a day. This number has been popularized as a standard goal, promoting a lifestyle that incorporates regular walking. However, this target may vary based on individual fitness levels and goals. Some people may find success with a goal of 7,000 to 8,000 steps, while others might aim higher if they are more active.
- **Breaking It Down**: To reach your step goal, consider breaking it down into manageable chunks. For example, aiming for 2,000 steps in the morning, another 2,000 during lunch, and then adding short walks throughout the afternoon can make achieving your goal feel less daunting. Use a pedometer or smartphone app to track your steps, providing motivation and accountability.
- **Incorporating Walking**: Integrate walking into your daily routine in simple ways, such as taking short walks during breaks, walking meetings, or even going

for a stroll after dinner. Every step counts, and these small increments add up throughout the day.

Incorporating Movement into Your Workday

- **Standing Desks**: If you have a desk job, consider using a standing desk or an adjustable desk that allows you to alternate between sitting and standing. Standing while working can help improve circulation, reduce sedentary time, and increase overall energy expenditure.
- **Active Breaks**: Schedule short breaks every hour to stretch, walk around, or do quick exercises like squats or lunges. Even a few minutes of movement can help combat the negative effects of prolonged sitting and boost your energy levels.
- **Walking Meetings**: If possible, suggest walking meetings with colleagues instead of sitting in a conference room. This not only allows for physical activity but can also promote creative thinking and enhance collaboration.

- **Find Activities You Enjoy**: Explore different forms of physical activity outside the gym that you genuinely enjoy. This could be hiking, dancing, cycling, or participating in community sports. When you find activities that are fun, you're more likely to stick with them long-term.
- **Set Specific Goals**: Create specific, achievable goals related to your daily activity. For example, aim to walk for 30 minutes each evening or sign up for a local sports league. Having clear objectives can provide motivation and help track your progress.
- **Make It a Social Event**: Involve friends or family in your daily activities. Plan group walks, play sports together, or take dance classes as a group. Making physical activity a social event can make it more enjoyable and encourage regular participation.

Summary

Creating a daily activity routine is key to boosting your overall health and supporting your weight loss efforts. By setting a daily walking goal, incorporating movement into your workday, and developing enjoyable habits outside of the gym, you can increase your daily activity levels and enhance your quality of life. Remember that consistency is essential—by making movement a regular part of your routine, you're more likely to achieve your fitness goals and create lasting, healthy habits.

Tracking your Physical Activity

Monitoring your physical activity is an essential component of any effective weight loss and fitness plan. By keeping track of your steps, calories burned, and overall activity levels, you can stay motivated, identify areas for improvement, and adjust your goals as needed. Let's explore the tools available for tracking your activity, the importance of consistency, and how to set realistic activity goals.

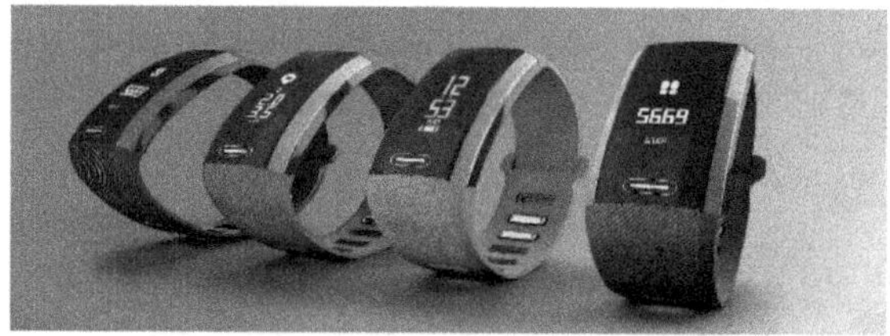

- **Fitness Trackers**: Wearable devices like fitness trackers or smartwatches are popular tools for monitoring physical activity. These devices typically track steps taken, calories burned, heart rate, and sometimes even sleep patterns. Many also offer features like reminders to move, which can help you stay active throughout the day.
- **Mobile Apps**: There are numerous apps available for both iOS and Android devices that can help you track your physical activity. Popular apps like MyFitnessPal, Fitbit, and Apple Health allow you to log your steps, workouts, and calories burned. Many of these apps also provide insights into your overall activity levels and progress toward your goals.
- **Manual Tracking**: If you prefer a more hands-on approach, consider keeping a physical journal or a digital spreadsheet to log your daily activity. This can include tracking your steps, workouts, and any other physical activities you engage in. Writing down your progress can help reinforce your commitment and keep you accountable.

- **Building Habits**: Consistency is key when it comes to reaping the benefits of physical activity. Regularly tracking your activity helps you establish healthy habits, making it easier to incorporate movement into your daily routine. The more consistent you are, the more natural it becomes to stay active.

- **Monitoring Progress**: By consistently tracking your activity, you can identify trends over time, such as when you tend to be more or less active. This insight can help you adjust your routines to stay on track with your fitness goals and recognize when you may need to increase your efforts.

- **Staying Motivated**: Seeing your progress can be a powerful motivator. Regularly reviewing your activity levels can remind you of how far you've come and encourage you to keep pushing toward your goals. Whether you hit a step goal or complete a challenging workout, celebrating these small victories can boost your motivation and commitment.

- **Start Small**: When setting activity goals, it's important to be realistic and achievable. If you're just starting, aim for small, incremental goals, such as increasing your daily step count by 500 steps each week. Gradually increasing your activity will help you build confidence and avoid feeling overwhelmed.

- **Be Flexible**: Life can be unpredictable, so be prepared to adjust your goals as needed. If you find that a specific goal is too challenging or doesn't fit your lifestyle, reassess and modify it. Flexibility in goal-setting allows you to maintain consistency without feeling discouraged.

- **Use SMART Goals**: When setting your activity goals, consider using the SMART criteria—Specific, Measurable, Achievable, Relevant, and Time-bound. For example, instead of saying, "I want to walk more," a SMART goal could be, "I will walk 10,000 steps each day for the next month." This approach helps clarify your objectives and makes it easier to track your progress.

Summary

Tracking your physical activity is a valuable tool for achieving and maintaining your weight loss and fitness goals. By utilizing fitness trackers, mobile apps, or manual tracking methods, you can monitor your steps and calories burned effectively. Consistency in your daily activity is essential for building healthy habits and staying motivated. Finally, remember to set realistic and adjustable activity goals to ensure your fitness journey remains enjoyable and sustainable. By taking these steps, you'll be well on your way to creating a healthier, more active lifestyle.

Chapter 5: Long-Term Success and Maintaining Weight Loss

Building Sustainable Habits

Creating a calorie-conscious lifestyle

Creating a calorie-conscious lifestyle is about finding the right balance between enjoying your favorite foods and making healthier choices that support your weight loss goals. It's essential to build habits that promote sustainability rather than temporary fixes. Here's how to strike that balance, develop meal planning routines, and avoid the pitfalls of "yo-yo dieting."

How to Balance Indulgences with Healthy Eating

- **Mindful Indulgence**: Allowing yourself occasional treats can be a crucial part of a sustainable eating plan. Instead of labeling foods as "good" or "bad," practice mindful indulgence. Choose your favorite indulgent foods and enjoy them in moderation. This approach can prevent feelings of deprivation and help you maintain a healthy relationship with food.
- **80/20 Rule**: Consider adopting the 80/20 rule, where 80% of your diet

consists of nutrient-dense, whole foods, and the remaining 20% allows for treats and indulgences. This flexible approach can help you satisfy cravings without compromising your health goals.

- **Portion Control**: When indulging, pay attention to portion sizes. Instead of having an entire dessert, opt for a smaller portion or share with someone. This way, you can enjoy the flavors you love while keeping your calorie intake in check.

Developing a Meal Planning Routine

- **Plan Ahead**: Meal planning is a powerful tool for creating a calorie-conscious lifestyle. Set aside time each week to plan your meals and snacks. This allows you to make healthier choices, avoid last-minute unhealthy options, and reduce food waste.
- **Create Balanced Meals**: When planning your meals, aim for a balance of macronutrients—proteins, fats, and carbohydrates. Include plenty of fruits, vegetables, whole grains, and lean proteins. This variety ensures you're getting essential nutrients while keeping your meals satisfying.

- **Prep in Batches**: Consider batch cooking or preparing meals in advance. This can save you time during the week and help you stick to your healthy eating plan. Prepare healthy snacks and meals that you can grab on busy days, making it easier to avoid unhealthy choices.

Practical Ways to Avoid "Yo-Yo Dieting"

- **Set Realistic Goals**: Avoid extreme diets that promise rapid weight loss but are difficult to maintain long-term. Instead, set realistic and achievable goals that focus on gradual progress. Aim for 1-2 pounds of weight loss per week, which is more sustainable and healthier.
- **Listen to Your Body**: Pay attention to your body's hunger and fullness cues. Practice intuitive eating by eating when you're hungry and stopping when you're satisfied. This approach can help you avoid overeating and promote a healthier relationship with food.
- **Celebrate Non-Scale Victories**: Instead of solely focusing on the number on the scale, celebrate non-scale victories, such as improved energy levels, better sleep, or increased fitness. Acknowledging these successes can

motivate you to stick with your healthy habits and reduce the temptation to revert to old patterns.

Summary

Building a calorie-conscious lifestyle is about creating sustainable habits that support your health and well-being. By finding a balance between indulgences and healthy eating, developing a meal planning routine, and taking practical steps to avoid yo-yo dieting, you can achieve lasting success. Remember, it's not just about what you eat but how you think about food and your relationship with it. With patience and persistence, you can create a lifestyle that promotes health, happiness, and harmony with your body.

Maintaining Physical Activity Level

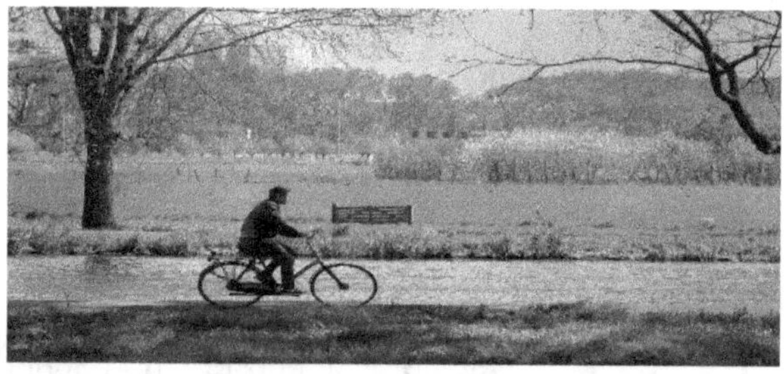

Maintaining regular physical activity is essential for overall health, weight management, and a vibrant lifestyle. The key to staying active is to keep your exercise routine enjoyable, incorporate active hobbies, and find a workout regimen that fits seamlessly into your life. Here are some effective strategies to help you maintain your physical activity levels for the long haul.

Keeping Exercise Enjoyable and Varied

- **Explore Different Activities**: To prevent boredom and burnout, try a variety of exercises. Whether it's dancing, swimming, hiking, cycling, or group fitness classes, experimenting with different activities can help you find what you love. The more you enjoy your workouts, the more likely you are to stick with them.
- **Mix Up Your Routine**: Incorporating different forms of exercise into your routine can keep things fresh. Alternate between strength training, cardio, and flexibility exercises throughout the week. Not only does this keep your workouts interesting, but it also ensures you're engaging different muscle groups and improving overall fitness.
- **Set Fun Challenges**: Setting personal challenges can add an element of excitement to your workouts. Consider training for a fun run, trying a new

fitness class, or participating in local sports leagues. These challenges can provide motivation and a sense of accomplishment that fuels your desire to stay active.

- **Incorporate Movement into Your Leisure Time**: Find hobbies that naturally involve physical activity. Gardening, dancing, playing a sport, or taking long walks with friends are great ways to stay active while enjoying your free time. This makes physical activity feel less like a chore and more like a rewarding part of your life.
- **Social Engagement**: Engaging in physical activities with friends or family can make them more enjoyable. Organize group hikes, join a community sports team, or attend exercise classes together. The social aspect can enhance your motivation and accountability, making it easier to stick to your activity goals.
- **Daily Movement**: Look for opportunities to be active throughout your day. This could include taking the stairs instead of the elevator, walking or biking to work, or playing outside with your kids. Small,

consistent actions can significantly contribute to your overall activity levels.

Finding a Workout Routine that Fits Your Life

- **Assess Your Schedule**: Take a close look at your daily and weekly routines to identify the best times for physical activity. Whether you're a morning person or prefer evenings, find slots that work for you and make them non-negotiable. Consistency is key, so aim for a routine that you can realistically maintain.
- **Be Flexible**: Life can be unpredictable, and it's essential to be adaptable with your exercise routine. If you miss a scheduled workout, don't be discouraged; find alternative ways to move throughout the day. A short walk, a quick home workout, or even stretching can help you stay active, even when time is limited.
- **Start Small**: If you're new to regular exercise, start with manageable goals. Aim for 10-15 minutes of activity a day, gradually increasing the duration as you build stamina and confidence. The most important thing is to create a routine that feels sustainable and fits comfortably within your lifestyle.

Summary

Maintaining physical activity levels is crucial for your health and well-being. By keeping your exercise routine enjoyable and varied, incorporating active hobbies and leisure activities, and finding a workout plan that aligns with your lifestyle, you can foster a love for movement that lasts a lifetime. Remember, the goal is not just to stay fit but to create a fulfilling and active life that brings you joy and energy. With persistence and creativity, you can make physical activity an integral and enjoyable part of your daily routine.

Handling Setbacks and Plateaus

Setbacks and plateaus are natural parts of any weight loss or fitness journey. They can be frustrating, but how you respond to them can make all the difference. By staying motivated, reassessing your calorie needs, and seeking accountability, you can navigate these challenges and continue moving forward. Here are some strategies to help you handle setbacks and plateaus effectively.

How to Stay Motivated when
Progress Slows

- **Shift Your Focus**: Instead of solely concentrating on the scale, celebrate non-scale victories such as improved energy levels, increased strength, or enhanced mood. Recognizing these achievements can help you maintain motivation and remind you of the benefits of your efforts beyond just weight loss.

- **Set New Goals**: If you find yourself plateauing, consider setting new, short-term goals to rekindle your motivation. This could involve trying a new workout, achieving a specific fitness milestone, or exploring a different healthy recipe. New challenges can reignite your enthusiasm and provide a fresh perspective.

- **Reflect on Your Why**: Revisit the reasons you started your journey in the first place. Reflecting on your motivations can provide clarity and encouragement. Whether it's to improve your health, boost your confidence, or feel more energetic, reconnecting with your "why" can inspire you to push through challenging times.

Reassessing your Calorie Needs and Adjusting

- **Monitor Your Progress**: Keep track of your calorie intake, activity levels, and weight changes over time. If you notice a plateau, it may be time to reassess your calorie needs. Your body's requirements can change as you lose weight or gain muscle, so staying aware of these fluctuations is essential.

- **Adjust Your Intake**: If you're not seeing the progress you desire, consider adjusting your caloric intake. Reducing your daily calorie consumption slightly or incorporating more physical activity can help reignite weight loss. Remember, small changes can lead to significant results over time.

- **Experiment with Macros**: Sometimes, tweaking your macronutrient ratios—such as increasing protein or reducing carbohydrates—can help overcome a plateau. Experimenting with different dietary approaches can provide insights into what works best for your body.

The Role of Accountability (Friends, Apps, Personal Trainers)

- **Find a Support System**: Surrounding yourself with a supportive community can significantly impact your motivation. Share your goals with friends, family, or join support groups where members encourage each other. Having someone to share your journey with can provide motivation and accountability during challenging times.

- **Utilize Technology**: Apps and online platforms can offer accountability through tracking and community support. Many fitness apps allow you to log your meals, workouts, and progress, helping you stay on track. Some even have built-in social features that let you connect with others pursuing similar goals.

- **Consider Professional Guidance**: If you're struggling to navigate setbacks on your own, working with a personal trainer or nutritionist can provide valuable insights and strategies. These professionals can help you create a tailored plan, offer support, and keep you accountable, ensuring you stay focused on your goals.

Summary

Handling setbacks and plateaus is an integral part of any weight loss or fitness journey. By focusing on motivation, reassessing your calorie needs, and building accountability, you can turn challenges into opportunities for growth. Remember that progress is not always linear, and what matters most is your commitment to long-term health and well-being. Embrace the journey, stay adaptable, and know that each step forward—no matter how small—brings you closer to your goals.

Building a Positive Relationship with Food

Maintaining a healthy weight is not just about calories in and calories out; it's also about nurturing a positive relationship with food. Developing a healthy mindset towards eating can help you overcome emotional triggers, view food as nourishment, and distinguish between true hunger and cravings. Here are some essential strategies to foster a positive relationship with food that supports long-term weight maintenance.

Overcoming Guilt and Emotional Eating

- **Recognize Triggers**: Understanding your emotional triggers is the first step in overcoming guilt and emotional eating. Keep a food diary to note when you eat for reasons other than hunger—such as stress, boredom, or sadness. Identifying these patterns can empower you to make more conscious choices.
- **Practice Self-Compassion**: It's essential to approach food choices with kindness rather than guilt. If you indulge in a treat or deviate from your plan, remind yourself that one meal or snack does not define your journey. Treat

yourself with the same compassion you would offer a friend who is struggling.

- **Find Alternative Coping Mechanisms**: Instead of turning to food for comfort, explore healthier ways to cope with emotions. Engage in activities such as journaling, exercise, meditation, or talking to a friend. These alternatives can help you process feelings without relying on food as a crutch.

Using Food as Fuel Rather than Reward

- **Shift Your Perspective**: Reframe the way you think about food. Instead of viewing it solely as a source of pleasure or reward, see it as fuel for your body. Focus on how different foods nourish and energize you. This mindset shift can help you make healthier choices and appreciate the role of food in your overall well-being.
- **Prioritize Nutrient-Dense Foods**: Fill your diet with nutrient-dense foods that support your health and energy levels. Focus on whole foods like fruits, vegetables, lean proteins, and whole grains. By prioritizing nourishing foods, you'll feel more satisfied and energized, reducing the urge to seek out less healthy options.

- **Mindful Eating**: Practice mindful eating by paying attention to your body's hunger signals and savoring each bite. This approach encourages you to enjoy the flavors and textures of your food, promoting a sense of satisfaction that goes beyond just fulfilling hunger.

Understanding Hunger vs. Cravings

- **Learn the Difference**: It's important to differentiate between physical hunger and emotional cravings. Hunger is a physical sensation that signals your body needs nourishment, while cravings are often driven by emotions or specific triggers. Take a moment to assess what you're feeling before reaching for food.
- **Pause Before Eating**: When you feel the urge to eat, pause for a moment. Ask yourself if you're truly hungry or if you're responding to a craving. This simple practice can help you make more mindful decisions about when and what to eat.
- **Create a Hunger Scale**: Develop a hunger scale that helps you assess your level of hunger before eating. Rate your hunger on a scale from 1 to 10, where 1 is starving and 10 is overly full. Aim to eat when you're around a 3 or 4 and

stop when you reach a 6 or 7. This strategy can help you recognize and respond to true hunger while preventing overeating.

Summary

Building a positive relationship with food is crucial for long-term weight maintenance. By overcoming guilt and emotional eating, using food as fuel rather than reward, and understanding the difference between hunger and cravings, you can cultivate a healthier mindset. Remember, it's not just about what you eat, but how you think about food. Embrace this journey with compassion and mindfulness, and you'll find that maintaining a healthy weight becomes a natural and enjoyable part of your lifestyle.

Setting Realistic, Flexible Goals

When it comes to weight loss and maintenance, setting realistic and flexible goals is essential for sustainable success. Perfectionism can often derail progress, while adaptable goals can help you stay motivated and aligned with your lifestyle. Here are some strategies to help you set achievable goals and celebrate your journey.

- **Embrace Imperfection**: Understand that perfection is unattainable and can lead to frustration and discouragement. Accept that there will be ups and downs in your weight loss journey, and that's completely normal. Instead of striving for a perfect routine, aim for consistent progress over time.
- **Focus on Progress, Not Perfection**: Shift your mindset to prioritize progress rather than perfection. Celebrate the small wins—like making healthier food choices or completing a workout—even if they don't lead to immediate weight loss. Each step forward is a sign of growth and commitment to your goals.
- **Be Kind to Yourself**: Practice self-compassion when you experience setbacks. If you indulge in a treat or miss a workout, remind yourself that one moment doesn't define your overall journey. Acknowledge your feelings and refocus on your goals without harsh self-criticism.

*Setting Goals that Adapt with
your Lifestyle*

- **Create SMART Goals**: Use the SMART framework—Specific,   Measurable,

Achievable, Relevant, and Time-bound—to set your goals. For example, instead of saying, "I want to lose weight," try "I will lose 5 pounds in the next two months by exercising three times a week and incorporating more vegetables into my meals."

- **Be Flexible**: Life is dynamic, and your goals should reflect that. If you encounter changes in your schedule or lifestyle, be prepared to adjust your goals accordingly. This flexibility helps you stay on track without feeling overwhelmed or discouraged by external factors.

- **Break Goals into Smaller Steps**: Instead of focusing solely on your end goal, break it down into smaller, manageable steps. For instance, if your goal is to lose 20 pounds, set weekly or monthly targets that gradually lead you to your ultimate goal. This approach allows you to celebrate achievements along the way, keeping you motivated and engaged.

Celebrating Non-Scale Victories

- **Acknowledge Other Achievements**: Weight loss is just one aspect of your health journey. Celebrate non-scale victories, such as increased energy levels, improved sleep quality, or the ability to perform daily tasks with greater ease. These accomplishments are vital indicators of your progress and overall well-being.

- **Track Milestones**: Keep a journal or create a vision board to document your non-scale victories. Record moments when you feel more confident, fit into a favorite outfit, or receive compliments from others. Reflecting on these achievements can provide motivation during challenging times.

- **Share Your Wins**: Share your successes—both big and small—with friends, family, or support groups. Connecting with others who understand your journey can amplify your sense of accomplishment and inspire them to celebrate their victories too.

Summary

Setting realistic, flexible goals is crucial for navigating your weight loss journey with confidence and resilience. By avoiding perfectionism, adapting your goals to fit your lifestyle, and celebrating non-scale victories, you can foster a positive mindset that supports long-term success. Remember, this journey is about progress, growth, and self-discovery. Embrace each step along the way, and enjoy the process of becoming the healthiest version of yourself.

Continuing to Educate Yourself about Nutrition and Fitness

In the ever-evolving landscape of nutrition and fitness, continuous education is key to making informed decisions that support your health and weight loss goals. Staying updated on the latest research and seeking guidance from reliable resources can empower you on your journey. Here are some essential strategies for ongoing learning in the realm of nutrition and fitness.

Staying Updated on New Research in Weight Loss and Nutrition

- **Follow Scientific Journals and Publications**: Keep abreast of the latest findings by subscribing to reputable health and nutrition journals. Websites like PubMed, Nutrition.gov, and the Academy of Nutrition and Dietetics offer valuable insights and access to cutting-edge research. This information can help you separate fact from fiction and make evidence-based choices.
- **Attend Workshops and Webinars**: Many organizations offer workshops, webinars, and online courses focused on nutrition and fitness. These events

often feature experts who share their knowledge on various topics, from meal planning to the latest exercise trends. Participating in these sessions can deepen your understanding and inspire new strategies to implement in your routine.

- **Stay Curious**: Cultivate a habit of curiosity about your health. Ask questions, explore topics that interest you, and seek out new perspectives. This proactive approach will help you remain engaged in your journey and open your mind to new ideas and practices.

Using Reliable Resources and
Experts for Guidance

- **Identify Credible Sources**: With a plethora of information available online, it's crucial to identify reliable resources. Look for information from registered dietitians, certified trainers, and reputable health organizations. Websites ending in .gov or .edu often provide trustworthy information backed by research.
- **Read Books and Articles from Experts**: Explore books written by nutritionists and fitness professionals who share evidence-based advice. Look

for authors who are respected in their fields and whose work aligns with your goals. Engaging with quality literature can enhance your understanding and motivate you to make positive changes.

- **Stay Skeptical of Trends**: Be cautious of fad diets or quick-fix solutions that promise rapid results. Often, these approaches lack scientific backing and can lead to disappointment or negative health consequences. A critical eye will help you discern between legitimate information and misleading claims.

Seeking Help When Necessary (Dietitians, Trainers, Coaches)

- **Consult with a Registered Dietitian**: If you're feeling overwhelmed or unsure about your nutrition, consider seeking guidance from a registered dietitian. They can provide personalized meal plans, address specific dietary needs, and help you develop a balanced approach to eating that aligns with your goals.

- **Work with a Certified Trainer**: A certified personal trainer can help you create a workout plan tailored to your fitness level and objectives. They can also teach you proper form and technique, which can enhance your results and reduce the risk of injury.

- **Consider Health Coaches**: If you need support with motivation and accountability, a health coach can be a valuable resource. They can help you set realistic goals, develop strategies to overcome challenges, and encourage you to stay on track.

Summary

Continuing to educate yourself about nutrition and fitness is essential for long-term success in your weight loss journey. By staying updated on new research, utilizing reliable resources, and seeking professional guidance when necessary, you'll empower yourself to make informed choices that support your health. Remember, learning is a lifelong journey, and the more knowledge you gain, the better equipped you will be to navigate the complexities of nutrition and fitness with confidence. Embrace this process, and enjoy the benefits of being an informed and proactive participant in your health.

Chapter 6: Closing

As you reach the end of *Burning Calories Made Simple: A Practical Guide to Effective Weight Loss and Transformation of Your Body*, I hope you feel empowered with the knowledge and tools to take charge of your health and well-being. Throughout this book, we've focused on providing a clear, fact-based approach to weight loss, helping you understand calories, and guiding you toward sustainable habits that fit your lifestyle.

Fight Weight Loss with Facts

When it comes to weight loss, there's no shortage of myths, trends, and quick-fix solutions that promise fast results. But lasting transformation is built on a foundation of facts. By understanding how calories work, the role of energy balance, and the impact of different foods and exercises on your body, you are now equipped to make informed decisions. Facts, not fads, are your greatest ally in achieving your goals.

Remember, this journey isn't about perfection—it's about progress. Weight loss isn't a straight path, and setbacks are part of the process. But with the right knowledge and a mindset focused on consistency, you can navigate challenges and continue moving forward toward your healthiest self.

Why Everyone Should Be Aware of Calories

At its core, weight management comes down to one simple truth: calories matter. Whether your goal is to lose weight, maintain your current body, or simply improve your overall health, having a basic awareness of calories can make all the difference. Understanding how your body uses energy, where that energy comes from, and how to balance your intake can be transformative—not just for weight loss, but for long-term health.

By becoming more calorie-conscious, you'll be able to make better choices for yourself, whether it's choosing nutrient-dense foods, practicing portion control, or maintaining a healthy balance between indulgence and discipline. This awareness is a powerful tool that can help you live a high-quality life, free from the frustration of constant dieting.

An Expression of Gratitude

Thank you for reading *Burning Calories Made Simple*. Your dedication to finishing this book shows your commitment to taking control of your health, and I applaud you for that. I hope the information, tips, and strategies shared here will serve you well as you continue on your weight loss journey or work to maintain the progress you've already made.

If you found this guide helpful, I kindly ask that you take a moment to leave a review on Amazon. Your feedback helps others discover the book and gives me the opportunity to keep improving and sharing useful content. I truly appreciate your support and would love to hear your thoughts.

Thank you again for joining me on this journey toward better health. Here's to making lasting changes, one calorie at a time!

ATHLEAN-X™. (2023, May 28). *The fastest way to get lean (FROM ANY BODY FAT LEVEL!)* [Video]. YouTube. https://www.youtube.com/watch?v=ZLmUDtbe1O8

BSc, K. G. (2018, May 11). *7 Proven ways to lose weight on autopilot (Without counting Calories)*. Healthline. https://www.healthline.com/nutrition/7-ways-to-lose-weight-without-counting-calories#:~:text=Eating%20Foods%20With%20a%20Low%20Calorie%20Density,content%2C%20such%20as%20vegetables%20and%20some%20fruits.

mountaindog1. (2019, August 9). *How to calculate your macros for optimal results "IIFYM"* [Video]. YouTube. https://www.youtube.com/watch?v=-Rc_C5L6QB8

Silva, S. (2024b, January 30). *Cardio or weightlifting: Which is better for weight loss?* Healthline. https://www.healthline.com/nutrition/cardio-vs-weights-for-weight-loss#takeaway